OPHTHALMOLOGY MADE RIDICULOUSLY SIMPLE

Stephen Goldberg, M.D.
Associate Professor
Departments of Anatomy and Family Medicine
University of Miami School of Medicine
Miami, Florida

MedMaster, Inc., Miami

I

Made in the United States of America

Published by
MedMaster, Inc.
P.O. Box 640028
Miami, FL 33164

ISBN 0-940780-01-1

TO SHAANI, RIVKA, MARC, AND MICHAEL

THE AUTHOR: Dr. Goldberg has a uniquely combined career as an ophthalmologist and family physician. A graduate of the Albert Einstein College of Medicine, he subsequently trained in neurology, ophthalmology, and family medicine, with board certification in the latter two fields. He is the author of *Clinical Neuroanatomy Made Ridiculously Simple*. In addition to direct patient care, Dr. Goldberg, as an Attending Physician in Family Medicine and as an Associate Professor of Anatomy at the University of Miami School of Medicine, is involved in the instruction of students and residents at a variety of levels. *Ophthalmology Made Ridiculously Simple* is a book for non-ophthalmologists, written by an ophthalmologist who views ophthalmology from the perspective of a family physician.

CONTENTS

Chapter

1 Anatomy 2

2 Visual Disorders 10

3 The Red Eye 22

4 Ocular Trauma 30

5 Retinal Disease 33

6 Neuro-ophthalmology 38

7 Ocular Findings in Systemic Disease 45

8 Ophthalmologic Techniques 49

    A.   Assessment of visual acuity. B. The direct ophthalmoscope. C. The indirect ophthalmoscope. D. Application of fluorescein strips and ophthalmic drops and ointments. E. The Schiotz tonometer. F. Assessing the depth of the anterior chamber angle. G. Removal of a foreign body. H. Securing an eye patch. I. The slit lamp. J. Cataract surgery.

9 Clinical Review 59

Glossary 78

Index 80

PREFACE

Most medical schools do not have a required course in ophthalmology. Consequently, students are often sadly deficient in this field unless they choose it as a specialty. In addition, a shortage of time prevents many from reading large texts on the subject.

This brief book focuses on that information most vital for the non-ophthalmologist. Many ocular conditions present first to the primary care physician. Included among these are refractive problems, ocular inflammations, trauma, amblyopia, strabismus, and a variety of additional disorders that cause diminished vision or ocular discomfort. It is essential for the non-ophthalmologist to know which problems to treat himself and which to refer. He must be sufficiently knowledgeable to detect subtle conditions such as amblyopia, which may be irreversible if not noted early and properly treated.

The book gives strong emphasis to common disorders, their diagnosis and management at the level of the non-ophthalmologist - up to the point of referral. Only minimal emphasis is given to the technical diagnostic and therapeutic measures that are the exclusive domain of the ophthalmologist.

Rather than text definitions of all potentially unfamiliar terms, a selected glossary follows the text. The clinical review in chapter 9 summarizes material already presented in the text, as well as miscellaneous other topics. The book also provides a rapid review for Medical Boards.

The attempts at humor in this text do not intend any disrespect for the field. They are employed as an educational device as it is well known that many of the best memory techniques involve the use of ridiculous associations.

I thank Drs. Cleve Howard, Fleur Sack, J. Lawton Smith, and Ronald Spielman for their helpful comments, and Beryn Frank for editing the manuscript. The cover illustration was prepared by Sixten Netzler. Text diagrams are by the author.

Stephen Goldberg

CHAPTER 1. ANATOMY

It is difficult to play billiards using eyeballs, as the eye is not perfectly spherical. The cornea is too steeply curved (fig. 1). This steep curvature enables the cornea to perform most of the refraction (bending and focusing) of light entering the eye. The cornea provides a coarse, nonvariable focus. The lens also focuses light, but only performs the fine variable adjustments. Contact lenses artificially alter the curvature of the front of the eye, thereby changing the focus.

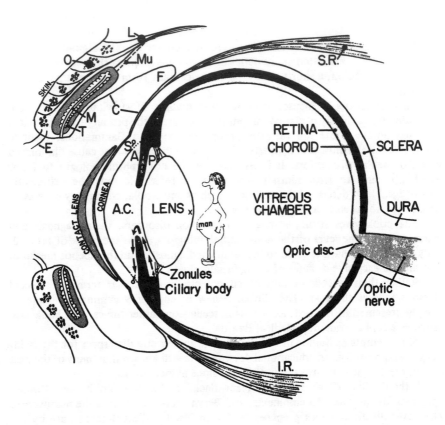

Figure 1. The eye. Arrows indicate the flow of aqueous humor from the ciliary body to the posterior chamber (P), to the anterior chamber (A.C.), to the angle (A), through the filtering (trabecular) meshwork (dotted lines) to the canal of Schlemm (S). A man in the eye is looking at the lens (see fig. 2). Most refraction occurs at the surface of the cornea. Contact lenses alter refraction by providing a differently curved surface with different refractive properties.

A, Angle of anterior chamber
A.C., Anterior chamber
C, Conjunctiva
E, Eyelash
F, Fornix
I.R., inferior rectus muscle

2

L, Levator palpebrae superioris muscle
M, Meibomian gland
Mu, Muller's muscle
O, orbicularis muscle
P, Posterior chamber
S, Schlemm's canal
S.R., Superior rectus muscle
T, Tarsal plate
X, A bad area of the lens to get a cataract

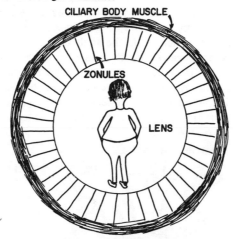

Figure 2. Rear view of the man in figure 1. Note that the muscles of the ciliary body form a ring.

Although only about 1mm thick, the cornea is tough. Following ocular trauma, its outer layer, the corneal epithelium (fig. 3), regenerates rapidly, with little scarring. Most trauma does not penetrate the tough Bowman's membrane that lies below the epithelium. Unfortunately, trauma that does affect the corneal stroma results in scarring. Particularly impaired vision results when such scarring involves the center of the cornea (in line with the pupil). Corneal transparency is based primarily on the geometric array of collagen fibers in its stroma. Damage to the corneal endothelium, which affects the water balance in this collagen meshwork, will result in corneal clouding.

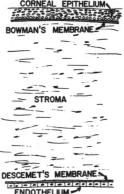

Figure 3. Layers of the cornea.

3

In some diseases, mineral deposits may settle in the cornea. The "poor" minerals (calcium, as in hypoparathyroidism; iron, from foreign bodies) tend to settle in "the Bowery" (Bowman's membrane). The "rich" minerals (copper, in Wilson's disease; gold, in gold poisoning, as in arthritis treatment; silver, following prolonged systemic or topical exposure to silver compounds) tend to deposit deeper, in Descemet's membrane.

The eye has three chambers: the anterior chamber (in front of the iris), the posterior chamber (between the iris and the lens), and the vitreous chamber (behind the lens). The anterior and posterior chambers contain the clear, watery aqueous humor produced constantly by the ciliary body. Aqueous humor exits the eye via the circular canal of Schlemm, which lies in the angle between the cornea and iris. The canal of Schlemm communicates directly with the venous system. Blockage of aqueous outflow results in increased intraocular pressure, termed *glaucoma*.

The ciliary body not only produces aqueous humor, but also contains a ring of ciliary muscles (fig. 2) that connect to the lens via fine, ligamentous *zonule fibers*. Contraction of the ciliary muscles affects the shape of the lens, thereby changing its focus - the process of *accommodation*.

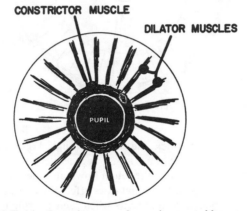

Figure 4. Muscles of the iris. Constrictor muscles are innervated by parasympathetic fibers of cranial nerve 3 (the oculomotor nerve). Dilator muscles are innervated by sympathetic fibers from the superior cervical ganglion of the neck.

The mechanism of accommodation is more easily understood through the mechanism of pupillary expansion (dilation) and constriction, as follows. The iris contains circular (constrictor) muscles at the pupillary border, and radial (dilator) muscle fibers (fig. 4). Note in figure 4 how contraction of the radial fibers would dilate the pupil. Contraction of the constrictor muscles decreases the circumference of the ring; therefore, the pupil constricts. The ciliary muscles, although more complex than the iris constrictor muscles, in a sense act similarly. Contraction of muscles in the ciliary ring narrows the diameter of the ring. This decreases the tension of the zonules, and releases tension on the lens. The lens then thickens (fig. 5), leading to a stronger focus (accommodation). Thus, accommodation is the process in which the ciliary muscles contract, thereby relaxing tension on the lens and enabling one to focus closer on an object.

4

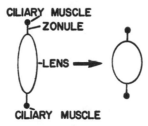

Figure 5. Constriction of the ring of ciliary muscles (see figs. 1, 2) narrows the diameter of the ring. This reduces tension on the lens. The lens becomes more convex and focuses the light closer to the lens (accommodation).

Opacities in the lens (cataracts) may obstruct vision, particularly when they are positioned centrally, in the posterior aspect of the lens (fig. 1). For optical reasons, cataracts in the anterior aspect of the lens or at the lens periphery tend to cause less visual loss.

The vitreous chamber contains vitreous humor, a thick gel. Unlike the aqueous humor, vitreous humor is no longer produced in the mature eye. Vitreous that is lost inadvertently from the eye during intraocular surgery cannot be replaced; fortunately, normal saline or aqueous humor may be substituted.

The eye has three main coats - the *retina, choroid* (a very vascular, pigmented structure), and *sclera* (the avascular "white of the eye"). After passing through the cornea, anterior chamber, pupil, posterior chamber, lens, and vitreous chamber, light then strikes the transparent *retina* (fig. 6). Light passes through the entire thickness of the retina before striking the photoreceptors (fig. 6). The photoreceptor cells initiate a chain of neuronal impulses from photoreceptor to bipolar cell to ganglion cell. The ganglion cell axons become the optic nerve, which extends to the brain (fig. 6).

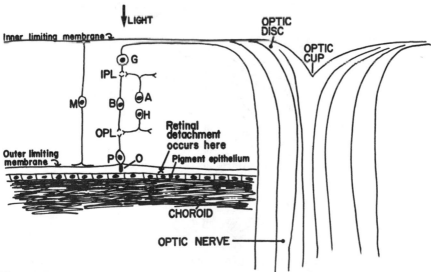

Figure 6. Layers of the retina (legend continued on pg. 6).

A, Amacrine cell
B, Bipolar cell
G, Ganglion cell
H, Horizontal cell
IPL, Inner plexiform layer
M, Muller cell
O, Outer segment of photoreceptor cell
OPL, Outer plexiform layer
P, Photoreceptor cell

Most of the retina receives its nutrition from branches of the central retinal artery, which lie within the retina. The photoreceptor cells, however, receive their nutrition largely by diffusion from the choroid. In retinal detachment, the retina separates from the pigment epithelium, a single layer of cells that lies closely adherent to the choroid. If not repaired within several days, the photoreceptors may be irreversibly damaged from prolonged hypoxia.

"Uvea" refers to the combination of the choroid, ciliary body and iris. All these structures are pigmented and continuous with one another. If one were to remove the sclera, one would note with great shock that the entire underlying eye, not just the iris, is pigmented. *Uveitis* is an inflammation of the uvea. It is "posterior" when the choroid is involved, or "anterior" when the ciliary body or iris is involved. *Chorioretinitis* is an inflammation that affects both choroid and retina.

Eye muscles

Figure 7 shows the anatomy of the extraocular muscles. Note that each muscle attaches to the eye as well as to some position on the *nasal* aspect of the orbit. None of the eye muscles attach to the temporal wall of the orbit. Keeping this in mind, you can appreciate the function of the eye muscles by imagining yourself pulling on each muscle in figure 7. The eye will move according to the scheme shown in table 1.

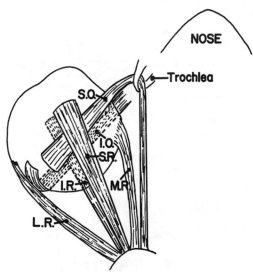

Figure 7. The extraocular muscles, viewed from above I.O., inferior oblique; I.R., inferior rectus; L.R., lateral rectus; M.R., medial rectus; S.O., superior oblique; S.R., superior rectus.

Eye Muscle	Nerve	Primary Function	Deficit
Medial rectus	Oculomotor (CN3)	Moves eye nasally	Eye is down and out because of unopposed action of lateral rectus and superior oblique
Lateral rectus	Abducens (CN6)	Moves eye temporally	Eye cannot look temporally
Superior rectus	Oculomotor (CN3)	Moves eye up	Weakness of upward gaze
Inferior rectus	Oculomotor (CN3)	Moves eye down	Weakness of downward gaze
Superior oblique	Trochlear (CN4)	1) Moves eye down when eye is already looking nasally. 2) Rotates eye when eye is already looking temporally. 3) Moves eye down and out when eye is in straight ahead position.	Vertical diplopia Head tilt (compensation for imbalance of rotation).
Inferior oblique	Oculomotor (CN3)	1) Moves eye up when eye is already looking nasally. 2) Rotates eye when eye is already looking temporally. 3) Moves eye up and out when eye is in straight ahead position.	Vertical diplopia Head tilt
Levator palpebrae superioris	Oculomotor (CN3)	Elevates upper lid	Marked ptosis
Muller's muscle (see Fig. 1)	Cervical sympathetics	Elevates upper lid	Mild ptosis

Table 1. Function of the extraocular muscles. CN, cranial nerve.

The orbital wall

The pattern of bones forming the orbital wall is shown in figure 8. The ethmoid bone lies near the nasal cavity. Following ethmoid fracture, infection can enter the orbital cavity. Air may also enter the orbit when the patient blows his nose, causing crepitus (a crackling sound) on palpating such an orbit. The floor of the orbit lies above the maxillary sinus. Orbital floor fractures may result in ocular misalignment when orbital fat and extra-ocular muscles become trapped in the fracture site.

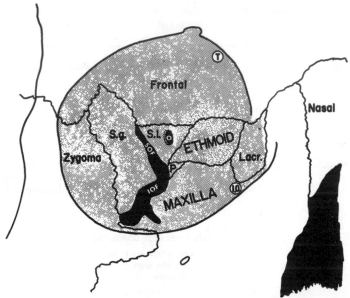

Figure 8. Bones of the right orbital wall, I.O., insertion zone of the inferior oblique muscle; IOF, inferior orbital fissure; O, optic canal; P, palatine bone; S.g., Sphenoid (greater wing); S.1., sphenoid (lesser wing); SOF, Superior orbital fissure; T, trochlea.

The optic nerve and ophthalmic artery (which gives rise to the central retinal artery) extend through the optic canal. All the other orbital nerves (cranial nerves 3, 4, and 6, the ophthalmic branch of CN5, and the sympathetic nerves to the eye), and the ophthalmic vein extend through the superior orbital fissure. Therefore, tumors of the optic nerve may enlarge the optic canal (visible on x-ray). Enlargement of the ophthalmic vein, as when it abnormally connects directly with the carotid circulation (a fistula), may result in enlargement of the superior orbital fissure and in compromise of the adjacent nerves.

Eyelids

The skin outside the eyelid is continuous, as a single sheet, with the lid and ocular conjunctiva, which in turn is continuous with the corneal epithelium (fig. 1). This continuity is fortunate; the folding back of conjunctiva in the fornix region (fig. 1) insures that a contact lens will not disappear behind the eye.

Each eyelid contains a firm collagenous tarsal plate which lends rigidity to the lids. This plate contains meibomian glands which contribute a sebaceous component to the tear film. An aqueous portion of tears is produced by the lacrimal gland, which empties into the supero-lateral fornix (fig. 9). Tear drainage occurs through the two nasally-located lacrimal puncta (fig. 9), which connect with the nose. Hence, one blows his nose when crying.

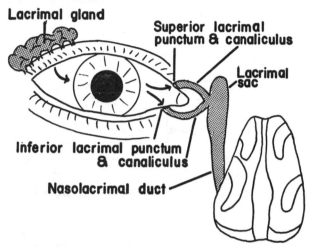

Figure 9. The lacrimal system.

An inflamed meibomian gland is termed a *chalazion,* which presents as a bump some distance from the lid margin. A *stye* is a pimple at the lid margin, resulting from infection of small glands in the lid margin (figs. 38, 39).

The levator muscle, innervated by cranial nerve 3, opens the eye. The orbicularis muscles (CN7) close the eyes (fig. 10). The levator muscle (CN3) opens the eye. The orbicularis muscles (CN7) close the eyes. This is not a misprint. The levator muscle (CN3) opens the eyes. The orbicularis muscles (CN7) close the eyes. This is a vital point in clinical diagnosis and therefore bears repeating. (see pg. 42 and fig. 58).

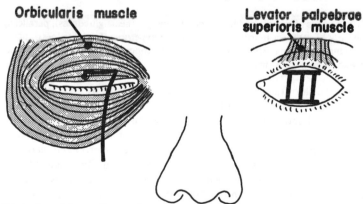

Figure 10. Action of the eyelid muscles. The orbicularis muscle (innervated by the facial nerve -cranial nerve 7 - a "hook") closes the eyes. The levator muscle (innervated by the oculomotor nerve - cranial nerve III - "three pillars") keeps the eyes open.

CHAPTER 2. VISUAL DISORDERS

If a camera is unfocused, focusing will help to sharpen the image. If the camera has a cloudy lens or damaged film, focusing will not help. Similarly, poor visual acuity may stem either from refractive errors (which may be improved by glasses - see fig. 11) or from non-refractive errors, e.g., corneal opacity, cataract, retinal detachment (which glasses will not correct).

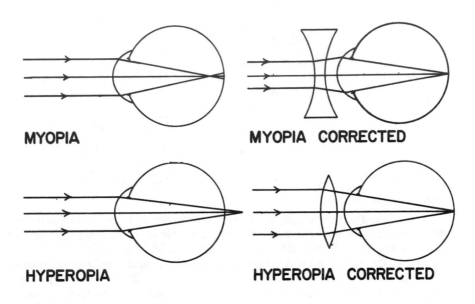

Figure 11. The optics of myopia and hyperopia. In myopia (nearsightedness), parallel light rays (from a distant object) focus in front of the retina. In hyperopia (farsightedness), parallel light rays focus behind the retina. Myopia is corrected with concave (negative) lenses. Hyperopia is corrected with convex (plus) lenses.

One can distinguish refractive and non-refractive problems by determining the visual acuity at far (via a Snellen chart, which is read at 20 feet away) and comparing it with that at near (via a hand-held Rosenbaum card - see fig. 12). The technique for testing visual acuity is described in Chapter 8, A. If near vision is good but not far, or vice-versa, the problem is refractive. Obviously, non-refractive problems lead to poor vision at both distances, just as a cloudy camera lens or torn film results in a poor picture regardless of the distance or focus. If vision is poor at both distances, the problem may be either refractive or non-refractive. Under such circumstances the nature of the problem may be uncovered either by testing lenses of various powers to determine whether they improve vision (a refractive error) or whether a pinhole improves vision (also a refractive error). The pinhole principle is illustrated in figure 13.

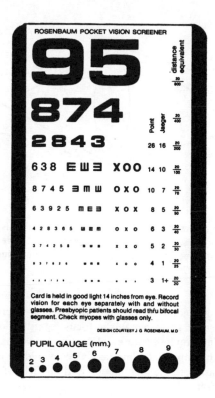

Figure 12. The Rosenbaum pocket vision screener, viewed at 14 inches. The Snellen chart contains similar, but enlarged, figures and is read at 20 feet.

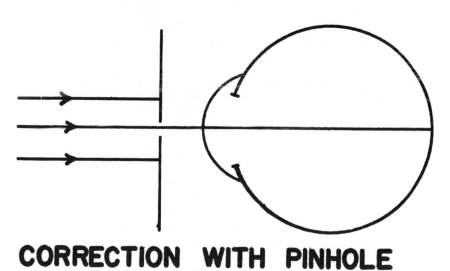

Figure 13. A simple pinhole will correct myopia or hyperopia.

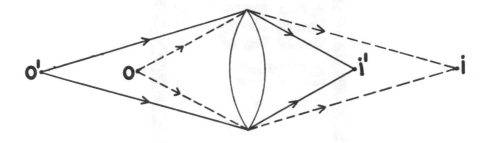

Figure 14. The closer an object (o) is to a convex lens, the farther is the image (i) focused. Hence, (see fig. 11) for myopes, near objects are focused closer to the retina than far objects and are seen best. For hyperopes, far objects focus closer to the retina and are seen best.

The pinhole restricts light to the center of the cornea, where refraction (bending of the light) is unnecessary. Light remains in focus regardless of the refractive error of the eye. The next time you lose your eyeglasses in the woods, try viewing through a pinhole; vision will be improved. Pinhole glasses would be used more frequently except that they decrease both the illumination and the field of vision, in addition to the weird cosmetic effect.

For clear vision, light must focus precisely on the retina. In nearsightedness (myopia: the patient sees near objects best), light is focused in front of the retina (fig. 11). In far-sightedness (hyperopia: the patient sees far objects best), light is focused behind the retina. Figure 14 illustrates why myopes have greatest difficulty with far vision, whereas hyperopic people have greatest difficulty with near vision.

Myopia commonly orginates in the young years as the eye grows. Typically a grade school or high school student experiences difficulty in reading the blackboard from far, or in seeing a movie from the rear of the theatre. The condition persists throughout life. Myopes always will require glasses (or contact lenses) to see distant objects clearly.

Hyperopia may be congenital. *Presbyopia* commonly arises and progresses from ages 45-60. Presbyopes have difficulty seeing near objects clearly, because this require accommodation; the ciliary muscle must contract, releasing tension on the lens, which then thickens. The lens becomes less resilient with age and does not thicken as readily; hence, near vision is poor in *presbyopia*. At first the patient may try to compensate for the low resiliency by trying very hard to accommodate, super-contracting the ciliary muscles. He may even be successful in this effort, but at the expense of inducing headache or fatigue. He may try to compensate by holding the newspaper farther away, wishing his arms were longer (fig. 15). Eventually, though, reading glasses become necessary to provide the additional focusing power.

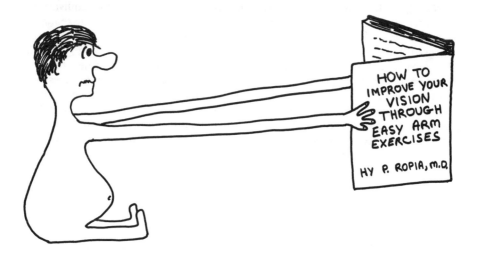

Figure 15. A presbyopic patient trying to improve vision by moving the object farther away.

The percentage of patients requiring glasses by age 60 in order to see perfectly for both near and far is close to 100%. The patient who never had a refractive error requires reading glasses as the eyes change between ages 45-60. The myopic patient may compensate for the need for reading glasses (plus lenses) by simply removing his myopic glasses (i.e., removes his negative lenses). However, he still, and always will, require glasses to see far.

The hyperopic patient who sees far well may never require glasses for distance. At some point he will require them for near, and at an earlier age than the patient who has no refractive error.

CASE HISTORY: Sam was a smart young intern. He always carried around a small Rosenbaum near vision-testing card (fig. 12) and routinely used it in his workups. The Rosenbaum card, of course, is the "equivalent" of the Snellen chart. Although the patient stands 20 feet away from a Snellen chart and only 14 inches from the Rosenbaum card, the letters are proportionately smaller on the Rosenbaum card to compensate for the patient being closer. One day, Sam became extremely perplexed. He had a patient with a cataract. The patient had 20/100 vision in the affected eye, whether using the Snellen chart or the Rosenbaum card. There was nothing unexpected about this; the near and far charts were "equivalent". Sam noticed, however, that his own vision (without glasses) was 20/100 for far (the Snellen chart), but an excellent 20/20 for near (the Rosenbaum card). "Something must be wrong with these charts," Sam thought. "I used good illumination and was the proper distance from the charts. I should have equal vision with either chart because the charts are 'equivalent'." Sam consulted his attending physician, who was not especially noted for keen judgement or knowledge. The attending tried the charts himself and, to his surprise, found that without his glasses he saw perfectly well for far but saw 20/100 for near, "Obviously", the attending commented, "these charts work only on patients." How does one account for these discrepancies?

ANS: Figure 16 illustrates why the Snellen and Rosenbaum charts are "equivalent". In order to see clearly, an image must not only be sharply focused on the retina but must be large enough. A microscopic object cannot be seen even though sharply focused. Patients may thus improve poor vision by using a magnifying glass. The Rosenbaum and Snellen charts are "equivalent" in that they both project the same sized images on the retina. In order to clearly see the letters, however, the eyes must focus them. The attending was presbyopic and had difficulties focusing for near. Sam was myopic. He saw perfectly for near but could not focus for far. Both Sam and the attending had *refractive* errors. The patient had a non-refractive problem; the focusing mechanism was working fine. The patient's problem was one of the cloudiness of the ocular media. One would expect his vision to be as poor for near as for far.

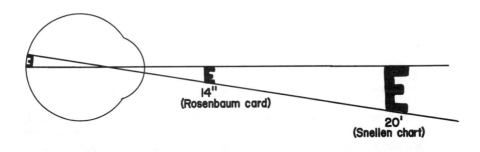

Figure 16. The basis for the equivalence of the Rosenbaum card and Snellen chart (see text for explanation).

QUESTION: Which method should the physician use for routine visual testing, the near chart or distant chart?

ANS: If one wishes to be certain that a patient has no difficulty in visual acuity, both near and far must be tested. Certainly, testing far vision alone is insufficient for the middle age patient who reports headaches, fatigue and blurred vision on reading up close. Near testing must be performed to evaluate presbyopia. Similarly, when a teenager reports difficulty seeing distant objects, near vision testing is insufficient. Sometimes, the physician is selectively interested in determining whether the patient has a non-refractive error (e.g., visual loss from acute ocular trauma). Under such conditions it may suffice to test either near or far vision as the finding of normal vision for either would rule out visual loss from such a condition. In general, it is best to test both near and far vision.

Astigmatism

A spherical lens bends light equally all around its circumference (fig. 17A). A spherical refractive error is erased by introducing a spherical lens of opposite refractive properties. A cylindrical lens bends light along only one axis as only one of its axes is curved (fig. 17B). A cylindrical refractive error (astigmatism) is corrected by introducing a cylindrical lens of opposite refractive properties. Patients may have a combination of astigmatism and a spherical refractive error. In that case the physician may correct the problem by combining a spherical lens with a cylindrical lens placed along the appropriate axis.

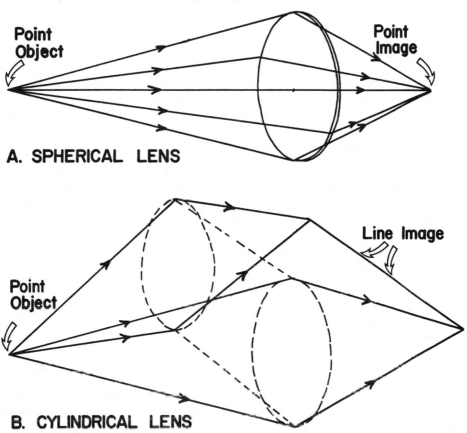

A. SPHERICAL LENS

B. CYLINDRICAL LENS

Figure 17. Optics of the spherical and cylindrical lens. For the cylindrical lens, a point object is focused as a line. An oval lens mathematically is a combination of a spherical and cyclindrical lens. In classic astigmatism, the cornea is oval. The eyeglass prescription is a combination of a spherical and cylindrical lens.

Reading Prescriptions

The following is a sample eyeglass prescription.

OD -2.00   +0.75 x 180°

OS -1.75   +0.25 x 180°   Add +1.50 ou

This means: In the right eye (OD) the correction calls for a minus (concave) 2.00 spherical lens, combined with a plus (convex) 0.75 cylindrical lens placed at an axis of 180°. The left eye (OS) requires a minus 1.75 spherical lens combined with a +0.25 cylinder at 180°. In addition the patient has difficulty with near vision (probably presbyopia) and requires for each eye (ou) a plus 1.50 spherical lens added on to the rest of the prescription as a bifocal segment, for near vision. The bifocal add is generally placed at the bottom of the eyeglasses as it is used when the patient is looking down, to focus on near objects.

Amblyopia and strabismus

Amblyopia is a visual disturbance with no apparent gross pathology. There is no cloudiness of the cornea or lens, or apparent retinal lesions. Amblyopia is not corrected by glasses. It is a microscopic defect in the wiring of the retina -to-brain connections that results from disuse of one eye at an early age (generally before age 7). An adult who does not use an eye will not develop amblyopia. A child below age 7 who does not use an eye will develop amblyopia, and the condition may become irreversible if not corrected quickly. Amblyopia occurs in only one eye. It is proposed that connections in the brain from one eye do not develop well if that eye is not used. Instead, connection sites are usurped by nerve fibers from the good eye. After maturity, correcting the cause of amblyopia will not restore function, as the connection (synaptic) sites are already filled by permanent connections from the normal eye.

There are three main causes of amblyopia - physical occlusion (as by cataract or ptosis), refractive errors, and strabismus. Strabismus, which affects about 2-3% of the population, is an abnormal turning of the eye either inward (crossed eyes; esotropia) or outward (wall-eyes; exotropia) If a child's eye has a refractive error, in effect that eye suffers from disuse and develops amblyopia. The treatment for refractive amblyopia is early correction of visual acuity.

Amblyopia caused by strabismus is also the product of disuse. A child with crossed eyes does not see double. Rather, he learns to suppress the vision in one eye to avoid seeing double. The suppressed eye, in effect, experiences "disuse" and becomes amblyopic. The initial treatment for strabismic amblyopia is to force the use of the eye by covering the normal eye. Correction of the strabismus is also part of the treatment. This sometimes requires surgery. At other times, particularly when the basis for strabismus is an overconvergence of the eyes on attempted accommodation (the eyes normally converge when acccommodating), treatment may be accomplished by accommodating for the patient. Glasses, or special eye drops (e.g., Phospholine iodide, a long-acting anticholinesterase) that constrict the ciliary muscles, are sometimes employed effectively. An adult who develops strabismus (e.g., from trauma) does not suppress vision in one eye, but sees double for the rest of his life.

When children with amblyopia wear a patch over the good eye, the eye with poor vision is forced into seeing and may improve. Surgery for strabismus generally has better results when both eyes see well. It is important to alternate the patch from one eye to the other, as amblyopia may be induced in the good eye by covering it for too many days!

Detecting amblyopia

The physician must be on particular lookout for the child with the potential of developing amblyopia. Otherwise, the child, once past the critical age of 7, will remain with a permanent defect in vision and never develop adequate stereoscopic vision. The proper examination consists in the determination of visual acuity in each eye and in assessing the child for strabismus.

If the child is too young to test vision with a Snellen or other visual chart, obtain the child's reaction to covering and uncovering each eye (fig. 18). If the child cries or fusses more when one eye in particular is covered, this is likely to be due to visual impairment in the eye being tested (the uncovered eye). The child becomes upset when the good eye is blocked.

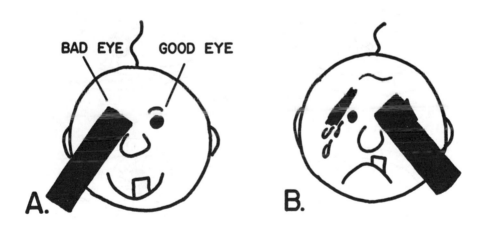

Figure 18. Assessment of a visual deficit in an infant. The child is disturbed when the well-seeing eye is covered.

17

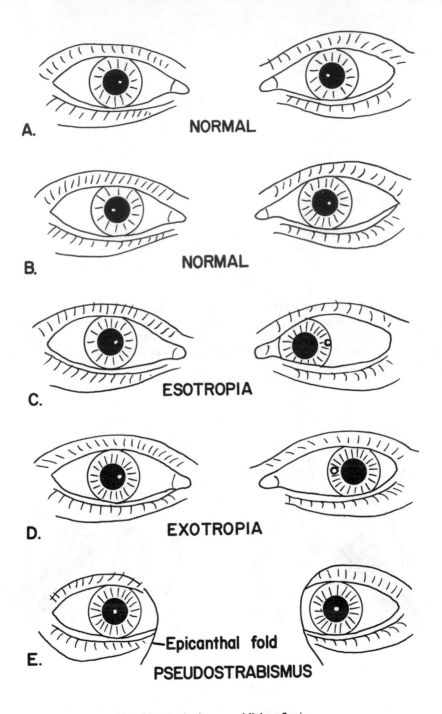

A. NORMAL

B. NORMAL

C. ESOTROPIA

D. EXOTROPIA

E. —Epicanthal fold
PSEUDOSTRABISMUS

Figure 19. Assessment of strabismus via the corneal light reflection.
  A. Reflection falls slightly nasal in each eye (normal).
  B. Reflection slightly temporal in each eye (normal—but refer anyway to check for strabismus).
  C. Characteristic asymmetry of the light reflection in cross-eyed strabismus (esotropia).
  D. Characteristic asymmetry of the light reflection in wall-eyed strabismus (exotropia):

One may assess strabismus by having the child focus on a small penlight held directly in front of the examiner's nose (fig. 19). If the pupillary reflex (seen as a pinpoint of light) occurs either dead center in each cornea, lateral to the center in each eye, or nasal to the center in each eye (i.e., a mirror image), these are normal variants; both eyes are aligned to the same degree with the object. Pattern 19B, however, should be referred anyway to check for strabismus, as it is very uncommon as a normal variant. If the image does not fall on each eye in a mirror image fashion, one eye is being used and the other isn't. Strabismus is present. If there is any suspicion of decreased visual acuity or strabismus, the child should be referred to an ophthalmologist for more subtle testing. An absence of stereoscopic (3-D) vision is also grounds for referral, as it may be due to amblyopia or strabismus. Stereoscopic vision may be simply tested. Have the patient hold a pencil in each hand at arms length and try to touch the points together. This is difficult to accomplish without stereoscopic vision.

Sometimes a child's eyes seem normal, but the mother says that at certain times during the day (not now), they appear crossed. What should the physician do then? This is a simple matter. The child should always be referred, because the mother is always right. The child is experiencing intermittent strabismus, often the result of fatigue, particularly at the end of the day.

QUESTION: Why do some children look cross-eyed, whereas examination for strabismus is normal?

ANS: These children have common, functional pseudostrabismus. In this situation prominent skin folds on the nasal aspect of the eyes (*epicanthal folds*) cause the artifactual appearance of strabismus (fig. 19E). Try simulating this on yourself. Look directly ahead into a mirror. Then, place a finger along each side of the nose, nasal to each eye. Your eyes will appear crossed, even though they are still looking straight ahead. With age, epicanthal folds decrease, and the child "outgrows" the pseudostrabismus.

Surgery for strabismus aims to realign the eyes. Various ocular muscles may be "strengthened" or "weakened". "Strengthening" is accomplished by removing a segment of muscle, thereby shortening it and increasing its tension. "Weakening" is done by cutting part of the muscle, or detaching it from its ocular insertion and reattaching the muscle more posteriorly, thereby loosening its tension. For example, to correct inturning of the right eye, the insertion of the right medial rectus muscle may be moved back (i.e., the muscle is weakened) at the same time that the right lateral rectus is shortened (strengthened) - a "recess-resect" procedure. Local injection of botulinum toxin may be useful as a muscle-weakening measure in strabismus.

Color vision

Defective color vision is a hereditary condition based on a defective recessive gene on the X chromosome. Therefore, it is far more common in males than in females, affecting about 6% of males and 0.6% of females. There are three types of color photoreceptors in the retina - red, green and blue cones, and the defect may lie in any of these. Most patients with color defects have difficulty distinguishing reds and greens. Rarely, the defect may involve difficulty distinguishing blues and yellows. Various color plate charts (e.g., the Ishihara or American Optical color plates) are used to detect these deficiencies. The tests consist of pictures of letters or numbers composed of various colored dots. Incorrect perception of the figures occurs with defective color vision.

Contact lenses

Contact lenses rest on the cornea and, depending largely on their degree of curvature (and refractive index), alter the refractive power of the front of the eye. Contact lenses have certain advantages over regular glasses.

1. Many people find them cosmetically desirable.

2. In cases where there is an irregular, corneal surface and difficult-to-resolve astigmatism, contact lenses provide a fresh, smooth surface and can readily erase many forms of astigmatism. Keratoconus (cone-shaped cornea) causes blurred and distorted images and may be treated with contact lenses.

3. In cases of very high refractive error (e.g., after cataract surgery, when very strong convex lenses are needed; or cases of pronounced myopia where strong concave lenses are required), eyeglasses would cause a significant magnification (or minifying) effect. Patients with thick post-cataract glasses may see clearly, but the environment appears greatly magnified. This may be difficult to adjust to. The field of vision is also restricted, as there is pronounced distortion when the patient looks through the edges of his glasses. The patient's eyes also appear magnified to the observer. Myopic patients with strong eyeglasses see the environment as smaller than normal and experience similar problems of distortion when looking through the edges of their glasses. Their eyes appear small and beady to the observer. The magnifying effect of eyeglasses is similar to that observed on looking through a magnifying lens. The object appears larger (or smaller, depending on the type of lens used) the farther the lens is held from the object. A contact lens largely erases this problem, as it abuts the eye. Patients who require cataract surgery (usually performed when cataract vision is 20/70 or worse) can minimize the magnification problem even further by having an intraocular lens implant at the time of surgery. An artificial plastic lens is substituted for the real lens inside the eye. Patients who have had only one cataract removed often cannot use cataract glasses, even though visual acuity may be perfect with glasses. The magnification effect causes the image in the operated eye to be larger than in the unoperated eye. This size imbalance is very disturbing to the patient. When a patient is a poor candidate for a lens implant or contact lenses, it is usually unwise to remove a unilateral cataract, unless the unoperated eye see 20/70 or worse. Otherwise the patient will come to favor the unoperated eye because of the size imbalance, and the operation will be worthless. For details of cataract evaluation and surgery, see Chapter 8, J.

The disavantages of contact lenses are:

1. They cost more than eyeglasses.

2. The eye can be damaged, if the lenses are not worn or inserted properly. The cornea may become scratched or infected, or subject to anoxia if the lenses are not removed nightly or do not receive proper care. These problems should diminish with improvements in extended wear lenses.

3. Many people find them uncomfortable to wear or hard to handle. Soft lenses are more advantageous than hard contact lenses in that they tend to be more comfortable. However:

1. They are more expensive than hard lenses.

2. They absorb chemicals, and greater care must be taken to insure their cleanliness.

3. They tend to mold to the shape of the cornea and are not effective with high degrees of astigmatism (greater than 2 diopters) or other marked errors.

4. Visual acuity may not be quite as good as with hard lenses.

Intraocular lenses (implanted at the time of cataract surgery) are convenient for the patient, who does not have to bother with the insertion and care of contact lenses. Such implants may present significant complications, however, if they become misaligned or dislocate. This may occur with faulty surgical placement or inadvertent dilation of the pupil (if the lenses are fastened to the iris at the time of cataract surgery). In addition, a small percentage of patients develop a retinal detachment following cataract surgery. It is difficult to examine or operate on such patients after a lens implant, if the pupil cannot be dilated. More recent procedures implant the lens behind the iris without affixing the lens to the iris. The pupil can be dilated following such procedures. The lens does not fall into the vitreous chamber because the biological lens normally has a posterior capsule that is left in place on removal of the cataract (an "extracapsular" lens extraction, in contrast to an "intracapsular" extraction, where the cataract is removed along with the lens capsule).

Radial Keratotomy

Radial Keratotomy is a surgical technique for the correction of myopia. A series of 4 to 16 radial cuts are placed around the corneal perimeter through most of the thickness of the cornea. This alters the curvature of the cornea and decreases the myopia. The technique presently incurs a risk of corneal perforation, incomplete correction of the refractive error, glare, and fluctuating visual acuity (the corneal shape may change with alterations in intraocular pressure). Long-term results are still under investigation.

CHAPTER 3. THE RED EYE

Apart from disorders in vision, the most common opthalmologic complaint is discomfort of some sort in the eye: e.g., itching, burning, irritation and pain. The history may be particularly revealing.

History

Marked itching generally signifies allergy. Acute onset of focal sticking pain suggests a foreign body. Deep, intense aching pain may be found in glaucoma, uveitis, optic neuritis, or in referred pain from sinusitis, vascular and tension headaches. "Burning", "irritation", "sand-in-the-eyes", or similar discomfort localized superficially suggests a local disorder of the lids, conjunctiva, cornea, sclera, or episclera. The superficial nature of the condition may be confirmed by its disappearance on application of topical anesthetics, e.g., proparacaine (Ophthaine), or tetracaine (Pontocaine).

Photophobia is not especially helpful as a localizing sign, as it may signify predominantly intraocular disease (e.g., uveitis) or extraocular disease (e.g., keratitis, conjunctivitis).

The eyelids

Both styes and chalazions (defined in chapter 1), are initially treated similarly, namely with antibiotic ointments and warm soaks. In general, the ointment should be administered directly behind the lid (Chapter 8D), as penetration through skin is poor. A variety of antibiotics are acceptable, including sulfacetamide, Neosporin (neomycin & bacitracin & polymixin), and Garamycin (gentamycin). Styes almost always resolve with such simple treatment. Chalazions often persist but may be removed by a simple surgical procedure (local anesthesia) when cosmesis is a concern.

It is important to distinguish styes and chalazions from basal cell carcinomas which, like styes and chalazions, may be found on the lid and are relatively common. A dimpled or ulcerated, pearly, firm appearance increases the likelihood of malignancy (fig. 40).

Xanthelasmae are soft, asymptomatic, yellowish lesions on the eyelids, particularly common in diabetes and in patients with hyperlipidemia. They are benign and may be removed easily, if desired for cosmesis (fig. 41).

Blepharitis (an infection of the eyelids - fig. 49) is characterized by redness and scaling along the lid margins, and sometimes by diffuse redness and swelling of the lids. In *cellulitis*, infection is rampant throughout the lid tissue and sometimes involves the orbit. Topical antibiotics do not have sufficient penetrability to treat cellulitis; systemic antibiotics are necessary. Orbital cellulitis should be treated vigorously; there is danger in this condition that infection may spread via the opthalmic veins to the cavernous venous sinus of the brain. Cellulitis commonly is a

22

secondary infection. The primary infection may lie in the sinuses, or other body regions, spreading via the bloodstream. The most common organism is *staphylococcus aureus,* although other bacteria, viruses, or fungi may be responsible.

The lacrimal system

Swelling, redness and tenderness of the nasal aspect of the lower lid may indicate *dacryocystitis:* an inflammation of the lacrimal sac (figs. 9, 45). Blockage within the lacrimal drainage system will cause tears to overflow the eye. Infection of the lacrimal sac can be detected by pressing on the lacrimal sac and observing mucopurulent material backflowing from the lacrimal puncta. If topical and systemic antibiotics do not cure the condition within several weeks, a surgical procedure may be necessary, involving flushing out the lacrimal system. When this is ineffective, a more definitive surgical procedure is necessary to construct a new passageway for the tears.

Infection of the lacrimal gland presents as a tender swelling in the upper temporal aspect of the upper lid, where the lacrimal gland is located (fig. 44). Treatment consists of warm soaks and systemic antibiotics.

Conjunctivitis (fig. 50)

When the eyeball itself is red, close examination of the distribution and appearance of the redness helps to narrow down the differential diagnosis. Note whether the redness is due to an actual dilation of blood vessels or to a patch of hemorrhage. A few drops of blood spread thinly under the conjunctiva are quite visible and may frighten the patient into thinking he has a serious ocular disorder. In reality, reassurance is all that is necessary for the occasional, non-painful, subconjunctival hemorrhage that is not accompanied by visual loss. Such hemorrhages may occur spontaneously, or secondary to trauma, and should disappear spontaneously within 2-3 weeks. If it occurs repeatedly, a bleeding disorder or excessive anticoagulation caused by drugs should be considered. Subconjunctival hemorrhages accompanied by pain suggest conjunctivitis.

Conjunctivitis may be bacterial or viral. Often, the two are difficult to distinguish on exam. They both may cause diffuse redness and irritation, or burning of the eyes, or be relatively asymptomatic. The presence of purulent discharge with much crustiness of the lid margins suggests bacterial infection; the eyelids stick together, and the patient has to pry his eyes open in the morning. Most opthalmologist do not bother culturing the eye as usually conjunctivitis is self-limiting and responds to a broad range of antibiotics (e.g., sulfacetamide, Neosporin, erythromycin, Garamycin), given as drops or ointment.

Antibiotics do not help viral conjunctivitis. When it is unclear whether the condition is bacterial or viral, topical antibiotics may be given empirically. These are less likely to cause side effects than are systemically administered antibiotics.

In a few forms of conjunctivitis, specific antibiotics are indicated. Gonococcal conjunctivitis, which is marked by profuse purulent exudates, responds best to systemic penicillin combined with topical broad-spectrum antibiotics. Penicillin is not recommended for topical use as adverse sensitivity reactions are common.

Gonococcal conjunctivitis in the neonate most commonly occurs within the first 5 days postnatal. Inclusion conjunctivitis (caused by chlamydia, a large atypical virus) most commonly appears between 5 and 12 days postnatal and responds best to topical tetracycline or sulfa. The most common cause of neonatal conjunctivitis is irritation by the silver nitrate drops used routinely for the prophylaxis of gonococcal conjunctivitis (Crede' prophylaxis). It appears 1 day after birth and clears rapidly.

Tetracycline, given topically or orally, is specifically indicated for treatment of trachoma (see Glossary), a chlamydial infection. Herpes simplex, when it affects the eye, classically appears as a dendritic ulcer on the cornea (fig. 47). It responds to topical antiviral agents: e.g., acyclovir, vidarabine. Antibiotic ointments usually are applied three times daily. Antibiotic drops generally are applied four times daily, but may be given more frequently. Antiviral agents may require hourly application of drops.

It is important for non-ophthalmologists to avoid administering topical steroids, whether used alone or in combination with antibiotics. They may help decrease redness of the eye, but are not worth their potential side effects. If the infecting agent happens to be herpes simplex (which can masquerade in a variety of forms), steroids may induce a corneal perforation. A fungal infection involving the cornea may be exacerbated by steroid preparations. Steroids are useful for uveitis, but this condition should be treated by the ophthalmologist, who has access to a slit lamp and indirect ophthalmoscopy (Chapter 8C, I), which are vital in diagnosis and followup.

Corneal injury

Corneal injury, whether by trauma or infection, may also present with accompanying conjunctival injection. Hence, the cornea should be examined carefully in cases of red eye. Fluorescein will outline areas where the corneal epithelium has been interrupted. (Chapter 8D).

There are two highly painful corneal conditions that commonly occur late at night, and will be readily diagnosed by the sleepy physician, if only they are considered. The contact lens syndrome occurs in patients who have worn their contact lenses for excessively long periods. The patient removes the lenses, goes to sleep and within several hours wakes up with severe pain, as the corneal epithelium has been damaged. The loss of a portion of corneal epithelium is confirmed with fluorescein and treated with an eyepatch, analgesics, and reassurance that the condition will disappear soon, generally within a day or two.

The second corneal condition is due to excessive exposure to ultraviolet light emitted by a sun lamp or welding arc. Such damage shows up as punctate staining on slit lamp exam. Without a slit lamp, the condition should still be highly suspect on history alone, particularly when the patient reports falling asleep under a sun lamp. The treatment is similar to that of the contact lens syndrome.

In scleritis (inflammation of the sclera) and episcleritis (inflammation of the connective tissue between the sclera and conjunctiva), vascular prominence often appears peculiarly confined to the lateral or medial aspect of the conjunctiva (fig. 53). It may coincide with systemic collagen vascular disease. The eye may be very painful. The condition often responds to topical or systemic steroids.

Glaucoma

In glaucoma, intraocular pressure rises, with subsequent damage to optic axons. There are two major types of glaucoma - open angle (chronic) and closed angle (narrow angle, or acute) glaucoma. Glaucoma arises after obstruction of the aqueous outflow in the vicinity of the canal of Schlemm (fig. 20). Narrow angle glaucoma causes a painful red eye with extremely high pressure (up to 60 mm mercury). Open angle glaucoma, which is far more common than narrow angle glaucoma, is painless, had moderately elevated pressures, and does not produce a red eye.

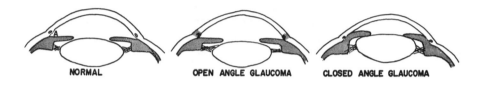

NORMAL   OPEN ANGLE GLAUCOMA   CLOSED ANGLE GLAUCOMA

Figure 20.The difference in angle (A) structure in open and closed angle glaucoma.

In narrow angle glaucoma, which constitutes about 5% of the glaucomas, the passageway for aqueous outflow is abruptly blocked by closure of the angle; the iris plasters up against the cornea (fig. 20). Dilating the pupils may bring on an attack, because the iris bunches up in the angle, which narrows the angle. In some patients, moreover, when the pupil is in the mid-dilated position, the iris comes into close apposition with the lens, thereby preventing aqueous humor from passing from the posterior to the anterior chamber. This builds up pressure, forces the iris forward, and contributes to angle closure. The only patients who are susceptible to angle closure attacks are those who normally have narrow angles to begin with. In such attacks the pressure rapidly rises, to perhaps 60 mm or more of mercury. It is not even necessary to use a Schiotz tonometer (Chapter 8E) to detect such high pressure. The eye becomes rock hard, whereas it normally has a slightly rubbery consistency. Since the attack almost always affects but one eye, the examiner can compare the hardness of both eyes by palpating each through the upper eyelid. Pain is intense; the cornea appears hazy; the patient sees halos around light, and there is a marked decrease in vision. Nausea and vomiting may be striking. The iris muscles become paralyzed, and the pupil becomes fixed in a mid-dilated position, unreactive to light. Blood vessels become especially prominent outside the perimeter of the cornea (fig. 51). If the attack subsides quickly, the pressure returns to normal levels, and the ocular exam is entirely normal except for the presence of narrow angles.

There are two key emergency measures to control the pressure chemically in an attack of acute angle closure glaucoma. One is the application of eyedrops to constrict the pupil (pilocarpine 4%, one to two drops every five minutes for 3 doses), which usually works within 20-60 minutes. The constriction serves in part to pull the iris away from the cornea, although the actual mechanism is more complex than this. In addition, oral glycerol (70 cc in 70 cc fruit juice on cracked ice) or intravenous mannitol (2 gm/kg.) should be administered. These are osmotic agents which draw water out of the eye and reduce the pressure. Once the attack has been broken, recurrence may be prevented by a relatively safe and highly effective procedure known as a peripheral iridectomy: a small piece of peripheral iris is removed, (or burned through with a laser beam) to allow a supplementary drainage route for aqueous into the anterior chamber (fig. 72A, B). Ocular massage has been reported to be a useful emergency measure in breaking an acute attack of angle closure. The chronic administration of pupillary constrictor drops has not been found satisfactory in preventing attacks of acute angle closure glaucoma.

In *open angle glaucoma* the blockage to aqueous outflow is more subtle, involving a microscopic blockage of aqueous outflow in regions near the trabecular meshwork and canal of Schlemm, rather than a gross mechanical obstruction by iris apposition to cornea.

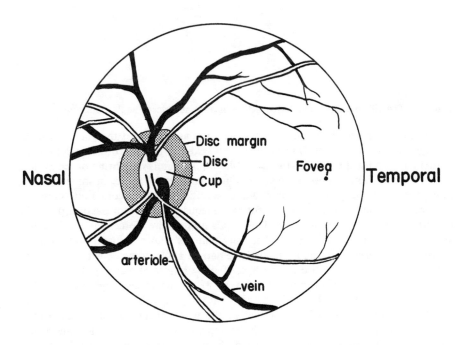

Figure 21.Schematic view a normal left retina. Note: The disc margin is well-outlined, disc color (shaded area) is a pinkish-white; the optic cup is a moderate size; four general groupings (arcades) of blood vessels spread to four quadrants of the eye; veins slightly larger than arterioles; no lesions; fovea lies about two disc diameters from the optic disc.

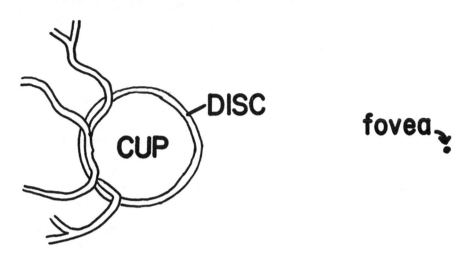

Figure 22. The optic disc in chronic (open angle) glaucoma. The cup is large and scooped out. The vessels are displaced to the nasal aspect of the cup. The disc is pale.

Unlike acute angle glaucoma, the findings in chronic (open angle) glaucoma are less dramatic, the product of only modest intraocular pressure elevation over a prolonged period. The eye is not red or painful; the pupil and cornea appear normal. Open angle glaucoma commonly affects both eyes simultaneously. The diagnosis is based on three points - the intraocular pressure, which normally should be less than 22 mm of mercury, is elevated; there are abnormal optic disc findings on retinal exam (figs. 21, 22); there is typical loss in the visual field exam. A pressure over 22, however, does not *necessarily* mean glaucoma, as it must first be shown that a visual field defect has occurred (figs. 24, 26). There are individuals with intraocular tensions over 22 who never develop glaucoma, as well as individuals with particularly sensitive eyes who will develop glaucomatous visual defects with pressures that are less than 22. Often the ophthalmologist, prior to instituting therapy, will carefully follow the patient's visual fields (e.g., every 6-8 months), and institute therapy at the first sign of a visual field defect. It is necessary to use a tangent screen or Goldmann perimeter (see Glossary) to detect such early visual field defects. The Snellen chart is inadequate, because the patient's visual acuity in open angle glaucoma characteristically remains normal until the disease is far advanced. While the peripheral field gradually shrinks, the fovea (the center of vision, which is predominantly responsible for good visual acuity) remains unaffected until the end stages of the disease. Roll up a sheet of paper and look through the tunnel. You will experience the constricted field of advanced glaucoma. Visual acuity remains perfect despite the constricted field. Open angle glaucoma is characteristically painless and is unaccompanied by a red eye or, in its early phase, by significant reduction in visual acuity. Therefore, it is incumbent on the general practitioner to screen for open angle glaucoma, which affects about 2% of the population over age 40, by direct retinal exam and tonometry. Tonometry (described in Chapter 8E) should be performed as part of the general physical exam in patients over 40, or younger if there is a family history of glaucoma. It should also be noted that there is an increased incidence of open angle glaucoma in patients who have diabetes, or who chronically take topical ocular or systemic steroids.

A further clue as to the presence of open angle glaucoma is the appearance of the optic disc on retinal exam. It characteristically is pale, with a large scooped out central cup and nasal displacement of the blood vessels (figs. 21, 22).

Open angle glaucoma is treated by drops that either dilate the pupil (e.g., epinephrine) or constrict the pupil (e.g., pilocarpine, or phospholine iodide). It seems strange that pupillary constrictors or dilators should help when obstruction by the iris is not the cause of pressure elevation. It is even stranger that dilators and constrictors, which have antagonistic effects, may be used simultaneously. Epinephrine acts by diminishing the secretion of aqueous humor by the ciliary body. Pilocarpine, in constricting the pupil, causes the iris to pull on the angle, and mechanically facilitates the passage of aqueous through the filtering trabecular meshwork. Oral medication, particularly acetazolamide (Diamox), may be added to the drops, if necessary. Diamox is a carbonic anhydrase inhibitor, and decreases the secretion of aqueous humor. Beta-adrenergic blocking agents (e.g., timolol) are also useful in decreasing intraocular pressure, possibly by decreasing aqueous secretion. Various studies indicate that marijuana may be a useful adjunct in decreasing intraocular pressure in open angle glaucoma, but is only effective for a short time before tolerance develops.

When medical treatment fails, surgery is performed. Although frequently successful, surgery does not have the same high success rate as in narrow angle glaucoma. An attempt is made to "unplug" the drainage system by incising the trabecular meshwork (via scalpel or laser beam). The eye may be opened to provide an artificial drainage connection between the interior of the eye and the subconjunctival space.

One commonly sees warnings in drug advertisements that a given drug is contraindicated if the patient has glaucoma. Such drugs may dilate the pupil and conceivably could cause an attack of narrow angle glaucoma. This warning is more to protect the manufacturer against unlikely litigation than for its practicality in a real clinical situation. The warning does not apply to patients with open angle glaucoma. Nor does it apply to patients with narrow angle glaucoma who have been successfully operated upon. Such patients are not adversely affected by the drugs in question. The drug warning applies specifically to patients who give a history of narrow angle glaucoma, and who have not as yet been operated upon. Such patients are exceedingly rare. If a diagnosis of narrow angle glaucoma had once been made, it is quite likely that the patient would have been operated upon. If the patient says he was not operated upon, it is likely that the "glaucoma" he refers to is open angle glaucoma, which is far more common than narrow angle glaucoma. You may suspect open angle glaucoma simply by noting the pilocarpine or epinephrine type drops that the patient uses. Even if one does cause an attack of narrow angle glaucoma, this will become immediately apparent through the patient's complaint of marked pain and visual loss, for which the treatment is highly successful (constrictor drops, osmotic agents and surgery). In fact, the patient may be fortunate to have the diagnosis made under controlled conditions where immediate medical attention is available.

Congenital glaucoma results from inadequate development of the filtering mechanism of the anterior chamber angle. Unlike adult glaucoma, the eye enlarges, as the young eye is distensible. Surgery is commonly indicated.

Uveitis

A *posterior* uveitis is an inflammation affecting the choroid, whereas an *anterior* uveitis affects the ciliary body (cyclitis) and/or iris (iritis). Uveitis may be caused by infection or allergy. Commonly the cause is unknown. The patient with uveitis, as in angle closure glaucoma, experiences ocular pain, photophobia, possible decrease in vision, and prominent blood vessels (injection) around the corneal limbus. Unlike the mid-dilated pupil in angle closure glaucoma, the pupil in uveitis goes into spasm and frequently is constricted (fig. 52). The eye is not hard and, in fact, may be softer than normal owing to decreased production of aqueous humor. The cornea does not look hazy as in angle closure glaucoma. The visual loss, where the retina is not involved, is due to haziness of the vitreous or aqueous humor, or to cataract formation. Such haziness cannot readily be assessed by the ordinary direct ophthalmoscope. A slit lamp is necessary (chapter 8, I). The latter contains a fine beam which demonstrates hazy fluid by the Tyndall effect (the reflection of light off suspended particles in a fluid - similar to the outline of a light beam shined through a smoky room).

It is important to dilate the pupil (e.g., with atropine) in uveitis, as the iris may otherwise become permanently stuck to the lens *(posterior synechiae)*. This sticking may obstruct aqueous entry into the anterior chamber and cause glaucoma. Topical, and sometimes retrobulbar and systemic, steroids are also employed to reduce inflammation. Uveitis should be followed by an ophthalmologist, as a slit lamp is necessary. Any patient with marked pain and visual loss in the eye, particularly if accompanied by a constricted pupil, should be referred for evaluation of uveitis.

A summary chart of The Red Eye may be found on the inside of the back cover (Fig. 72B)

CHAPTER 4. OCULAR TRAUMA

Blunt trauma

Don't press on the eye! When a patient with blunt trauma presents with swollen-shut lids, don't press on the eye! If you do, and the eye happens to be perforated, you will witness the squashed grape effect - the contents of the eye being extruded onto the cheek. A perforated globe can often be saved with proper suturing. Don't press on the eye!

In evaluating the patient with swollen-shut lids, first try to assess visual acuity. In order to do this, it may be necessary to gently pry the lids open and possibly apply anesthetic drops to reduce reflex tightening of the lids (but don't press on the eye!).

If the vision is normal or reduced only about a line on the vision chart following blunt trauma, most likely the globe is not perforated, as vision in most cases would be greatly reduced. Markedly reduced vision, in itself, however, does not necessarily mean a perforated globe. E.g., there could be a corneal abrasion, lens dislocation or retinal tear.

Check for diplopia (double vision) by having the patient follow your finger over horizontal and vertical excursions. If the patient reports double vision, confirm that it disappears on covering either of the eyes. If it does disappear, there is true diplopia and the eyes are misaligned. A nerve to an extraocular muscle, or the muscle itself, has been damaged, or the globe has been displaced due to tissue swelling or orbital floor fracture. In orbital floor fractures, the inferior rectus or inferior oblique muscle often becomes entrapped in the fracture site. The patient experiences particular difficulty elevating the globe. There may be anesthesia of the lower lid region from damage to the infraorbital nerve which runs in the orbital floor. Any sign of diplopia following injury should prompt an x-ray with orbital floor views to check for fracture. Cloudiness of the maxillary sinus is commonly seen accompanying orbital floor fracture and is caused by hemorrhage or prolapse of orbital fat into the sinus. Severe fractures may require surgical repair.

If diplopia does not disappear on covering the normal eye, it originates not in an imbalance between the two eyes, but inside the affected eye itself. There may be a dislocation of the lens. Alternatively, as occurs with many patients, the patient may say "double vision" but simply mean "blurred" vision.

Check the lids for swelling and laceration. Gently palpation of the swollen lids (don't press on the eye) may reveal a crackling sound (crepitus), indicating air within the orbit. This results from fracture of the thin ethmoid bone that separates the nasal passages from the orbit.

Look at the conjunctiva. Conjunctival lacerations generally can be left alone, as they heal well. Subconjunctival hemorrhages generally disappear spontaneously within 2-3 weeks. Check the cornea for cloudiness and signs of corneal abrasion or embedded foreign body. Flourescein will assist in detecting subtle corneal lesions. Most corneal abrasions heal completely within several days. Injury with wood or other plant materials, however, often are slow in healing. Examine the anterior chamber for a blood level (fig. 48), termed a *hyphema,* as opposed to a *hypopyon* which is a level of whitish inflammatory cells in the anterior chamber.

Check the pupillary size. Are the pupils asymmetric in size? Does the pupil in the affected eye respond to light? Is it distorted or displaced, suggesting intraocular trauma? Try to assess the depth of the anterior chamber. It may collapse in perforating injuries with aqueous humor leakage. Figure 35 illustrates a simple technique for assessing the depth of the anterior chamber. Can you visualize the retina well? Look for retinal hemorrhages or tears.

Refer to an ophthalmologist for signs suspicious of intraocular trauma - marked decrease in vision, shallow anterior chamber, distorted, displaced, or asymmetric pupils (▶ 20% difference in diameter is abnormal) or evidence of retinal damage, or ocular misalignment.

The general rule of "ice the first day and heat the next" applies to the eye, as well as to trauma in other areas of the body.

Lid and eyebrow lacerations may be sutured similarly to other body regions, except when the lid injury is deep or when the lid margins are involved. The latter situations require special surgical closures and are best referred. This is particularly true of lacerations in the vicinity of the lacrimal punctum, where improper closure may lead to a block in tear outflow.

In cases of severe ocular trauma, where the eye is lacerated and all vision is lost, the decision may be made to remove the injured eye, to prevent the possibility of *sympathetic ophthalmia* developing in the opposite eye. In this condition, the injury induces a type of autoimmune reaction which may cause blindness in the uninjured eye. Fortunately, this complication is rare. The surgeon and patient may be faced with a difficult decision, as to whether to remove the injured eye or to risk leaving it in for better cosmesis.

One other thing - don't press on the eye!

Chemical burns

There are two main kinds of chemical burns - those in which everything will be O.K. and those which are disasters. It is generally possible to instantly determine the prognosis.

In the more favorable situations the cornea appears clear. Fluorescein staining may show diffuse epithelial damage, but the epithelium heals very rapidly. A cornea totally denuded of epithelium may heal within several days. The clear cornea suggests that the stroma has not been damaged.

The disastrous situation is the white, opaque cornea, which signifies irreversible stromal damage. Corneal transplantation may be necessary, but often has poor results in severely burned eyes. Generally, alkalis (e.g., lye) are more damaging to the eye than are acids, although concentrations are also critical.

The initial treatment for both acid and alkali burns is profuse irrigation with water or saline for 15-20 minutes. Do not attempt to neutralize acid with alkali and vice-versa as is done with gastric poisoning. The heat of such reactions may further damage the eye. Look for pupillary constriction, a sign of irritation inside the eye. A slit lamp exam will detect cloudiness inside the anterior chamber with intraocular inflammation. If signs of intraocular irritation are present, cycloplegic drops may be beneficial. Aside from easing the patient's discomfort by relieving spasm of iris and ciliary body, cycloplegic drops dilate the pupil and pull the iris away from the lens, thereby preventing the iris from sticking to the lens and causing glaucoma.

31

Referral is indicated for signs of intraocular or marked extraocular irritation. It is necessary to follow the patient until the corneal epithelium heals over and intraocular inflammation subsides. Topical antibiotics and eye patching may be useful during the course of epithelial healing. Do not use steroids when there is any break in the corneal epithelium. They may predispose to complications from herpes simplex or fungal infection of the cornea.

CHAPTER 5. RETINAL DISEASE

Many diseases that affect blood vessels throughout the body also affect retinal vessels. The cornea provides a window in the body to observe various vascular diseases.

Hypertension (Figs. 23, 71A)

The severity of vascular damage from hypertension depends partly on the level of hypertension, and partly on how long it has been present. The degree of damage is apparently also dependent on the patient, as certain individuals appear more prone to vascular damage than others.

Certain hypertensive changes in the fundus relate to the *height* of hypertension (termed acute changes) and may occur immediately, if the blood pressure is very high. Other changes are chronic and may take years to develop (fig. 23).

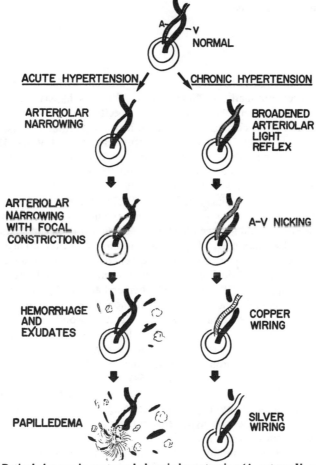

Figure 23. Retinal changes in acute and chronic hypertension (A, artery; V, vein).

Acute changes are the result of general and focal arteriolar constriction (fig. 23), possibly representing an increase in muscle tone. The arterioles appear narrow and tortuous. Ischemia and vascular permeability occur. Damaged optic axons swell in the local area of damage, forming soft, fluffy "cotton wool" exudates (fig. 23). Seepage of red blood cells and hemorrhages occur. Such hemorrhages commonly are "feathery" or "flame-shaped"; they outline the optic fibers that extend toward the optic disc (fig. 23). When hypertension is severe, the optic disc (papilla) may become edematous and surrounded by hemorrhages and exudates (papilledema). Although different stages have been assigned to these processes, it is perhaps more important to simply describe what is observed rather than assign confusing stage classifications.

Chronic hypertension also affects the arterioles, but differently than in acute hypertensive retinopathy. The arteriolar media (the central layer of the arteriole) thickens, thus gradually obscuring visualization of the blood through the normally transparent vascular wall. The normal arteriolar light reflection at first broadens (fig. 23). As the arteriole thickens, it presses on veins at sites where artery and vein cross, causing arteriovenous (A/V) nicking. With further thickening the arteriole changes color, producing "copper wiring" and finally "silver wiring", in which the blood column is totally obscured.

Diabetes

Diabetic retinopathy (fig. 69) proceeds by a totally different mechanism than the hypertensive retinopathy outlined above. Whereas hypertension affects the arterioles, diabetes affects the veins - more specifically the venous side of the capillary bed, as a venous occlusive disease. In fact, the picture in retinal vein occlusion may resemble that in diabetes. Classic findings are as follows: 1) The veins become dilated. Hence, there is A/V nicking in diabetes as well as in chronic hypertension. In diabetes, the A/V nicking stems from venous dilation, whereas in chronic hypertension it stems from arteriolar thickening. 2) Microaneurysms appear on the venous side of the capillary bed in diabetes, as areas of weakness and expansion of the vessel wall. These appear as pinpoint reddish spots, commonly surrounding the foveal region and may be difficult to distinguish from tiny ("dot") hemorrhages. 3) Retinal venules normally lie deeper in the retina than do arterioles. As a result hemorrhages in diabetes, a venous disease, tend to be situated relatively deep in the retina, as roundish "dot" or larger "blot" hemorrhages. These hemorrhages differ from the superficial "flame-shaped" hemorrhages of hypertension, which is an arteriolar disease. 4) Exudates in diabetic retinopathy also tend to lie deeper than those in hypertension. Whereas superficial "cotton wool" exudates are more characteristic of hypertension, the deeper lying, roundish "hard exudates", representing products of cell damage, are more characteristic of diabetes. 5) In diabetes, blood vessels may proliferate as fine networks of *neovascularization,* which can extend into the vitreous and bleed (fig. 69).

Commonly, diabetic and arteriosclerotic changes are found concurrently; hence, the frequent difficulty in precisely defining the etiology of the underlying pathology. In both diabetes and hypertension there are hemorrhages, exudates, and A/V nicking, but for different reasons.

Treatment in diabetic and hypertensive retinopathy consists of control of blood glucose and blood pressure. In diabetic retinopathy, laser photocoagulation may be applied to microaneurysms and neovascular areas, in selected cases. The laser beam is a form of intense, pure (coherent) light that can generate intense heat in pinpoint areas. When focused on the retina, laser light can eliminate microaneurysms and small, leaky blood vessels. The main complications of laser photocoagulation are inadvertent hemorrhage, and damage to critically important foveal fibers. Laser photocoagulation is performed as an outpatient procedure under local anesthesia.

The primary care physician should dilate the pupils and examine the retina yearly in diabetics without evidence of retinopathy. If retinopathy is present, followup should be performed by an ophthalmologist. The followup interval will depend upon the severity of the condition and the treatment.

Diabetic retinopathy is the leading cause of blindness in the United States. Trachoma, a chlamydial infection that causes corneal scarring, is the leading cause of blindness in the world. Trachoma is very uncommon in the United States except among American Indians.

Papilledema (fig. 63)

Increased intracranial pressure is reflected at the optic nerve head as venous obstruction. As a result, the veins and capillaries dilate in the region of the optic disc and give the disc an "angry" appearance. Extrusion of blood components results in disc edema, exudates and hemorrhage. Edema causes the disc to become elevated; the disc margins become blurred, and the central optic cup of the disc decreases in diameter. One of the first things to occur in papilledema is loss of the normal venous pulsation that occurs in the region of the optic cup. Such pulsation can be detected in most normal individuals. If the patient lacks venous pulsation, this tells you little, as venous pulsation may be difficult to detect in normal individuals. If the patient *has* venous pulsation, this is significant; it tells you that papilledema most likely is not present.

Even a single small hemorrhage or exudate is a strong sign of disc pathology, and may be due to papilledema. Disc elevation and small cup size are, alone, not reliable signs of papilledema, as they can be found normally. However, if these findings are asymmetrical, being present in one eye but not the other, suspect pathology. Disc elevation may best be detected by noting the tortuosity of the retinal vessels near the disc as they curve to go up and over the "hill".

If blurring of the disc margin is noted, determine whether everything is blurred, as may occur with a cataract, or whether the disc area in particular is blurred, as occurs in papilledema.

Surprisingly, the patient's visual acuity typically does not change significantly with papilledema. This contrast with papillitis, a much less common condition in which there is an actual inflammation of the optic disc that looks just like papilledema. Such patients experience a profound drop in visual acuity and, very commonly, marked eye pain that is deeply situated.

The hemorrhages and exudates in papilledema tend to cluster around the optic nerve head. This contrasts with the hemorrhages and exudates in advanced hypertensive retinopathy which scatter more broadly, throughout the entire posterior pole of the eye, including the optic disc.

The papilledematous disc, in a sense, looks like the reverse of the glaucomatous disc. In papilledema, the pressure is elevated outside the eye, in glaucoma, inside the eye. In papilledema, the disc is angry with dilated blood vessels and is elevated, with a small cup. In glaucoma, the disc is pale and depressed, containing a large scooped out optic cup (fig. 22).

Fluorescein angiography

In fluorescein angiography, an arm vein is injected with a fluorescein contrast material that is photographed as it passes through the retinal vessels. The technique is extremely useful in outlining a variety of conditions. If there is a question as to whether or not papilledema or papillitis is present, fluorescein angiography will reveal fluorescein leakage around the optic disc in either of these conditions. No leakage occurs normally. In diabetic retinopathy, the technique will detect many more microaneurysms than can be seen with the ophthalmoscope. Delimiting the areas of leakage from microaneurysms and neovascularization helps determine the areas to attack with laser photocoagulation in diabetic retinopathy. Fluorescein leakage patterns may help distinguish choroidal melanomas and other malignant tumors (fig. 61) from benign conditions. Further confirmation of the presence of a melanoma can be obtained by noting with special probes the propensity of melanomas to concentrate injected radioactive P32.

Retinal detachment (fig. 65)

In retinal detachment, fluid collects between the retina and the pigment epithelium. In a partial detachment the patient commonly reports floaters, flashes of light, and the sensation of a dense curtain being drawn partially over the eyes. Since the photoreceptor layer of the retina receives its oxygenation via diffusion from the choroid, the separation of the retina adversely affects the photoreceptor layer in particular. If not repaired surgically within several days, the damage may be irreversible.

The surgeon attempts to reattach the retina and pigment epithelium under general anesthesia. The techniques may involve draining subretinal fluid with a fine needle passed through the sclera; rendering the pigment epithelium more sticky by applying an intensely cold probe (a cryoprobe) to the sclera near the site of detachment; indenting the sclera with a special buckle affixed outside the eye so as to mechanically push the pigment epithelium against the retina. In selected cases laser photocoagulation may be used to seal holes in the retina (under local anesthesia). Retinal holes predispose to retinal detachment by allowing fluid to leak from the vitreous chamber to the space between the retina and pigment epithelium.

Retinal detachment and retinal degeneration are more common in myopes than in patients with other types of refractive errors. Detachments are much more common following cataract surgery or severe ocular injury.

Macular degeneration (Fig. 66)

The fovea (fig. 21), a pinpoint, depressed area of the central retina, is the retinal area with greatest visual acuity. This area plus the area surrounding it is termed the macula. Macular degeneration is the leading cause of blindness in the elderly. It may also occur in children and young adults as a hereditary disorder. The patient experiences great difficulty in reading and often must resort to a magnifying glass, as a magnified image occupies a broad span of retina, including areas that have been unaffected by the disease. The peripheral retina is usually spared. Although the person is "legally blind", he or she is rarely "cane-tapping blind", and gets about quite well. Reading and driving abilities are the major loss. Sometimes macular degeneration is amenable to laser photocoagulation - when fluorescein angiography reveals leakage of fluid under the retina. If the leak is not directly in the center of the macula, laser treatment may be useful in sealing the leak.

Sometimes, it is difficult to assess the degree to which a patient's visual loss is due to macular degeneration, and the degree to which cataracts are responsible. Both may coexist. One would not want to remove the cataract if the visual problem is due to macular degeneration. A useful rule is: "If the examiner can see in, the patient can see out." I.e., if the examiner can see the retina clearly using the ophthalmoscope, it is unlikely that the cataract is sufficiently dense to cause a significant problem in visual acuity.

Retinitis pigmentosa

In retinitis pigmentosa the retina contains areas of peppery or bone-spicule pigmentary degeneration, often in a circular distribution (fig. 64). Such patients experience particular difficulty with night vision in this hereditary degenerative disease. Presently there is no satisfactory treatment.

Retinitis pigmentosa should be distinguished from old chorioretinitis. It is not uncommon to find a solitary patch of pigmentary degeneration during a routine retinal exam, which typically signifies an old, inactive chorioretinitis (fig. 60).

Retrolental fibroplasia

Retrolental fibroplasia is a vascular proliferative disease of the retina. It stems from excessive administration of oxygen to premature infants. Vascularization may spread to the vitreous with subsequent vitreous scarring, retinal detachment, and blindness. Unfortunately, the prognosis in advanced cases is presently unfavorable, even in the best surgical hands.

Retinoblastoma

Retinoblastoma is a congenital malignant retinal tumor. It may occur sporadically or be transmitted as an autosomal dominant gene with incomplete penetrance. The child commonly presents with a white pupil. One or both eyes may be affected. Treatment is removal of the eye (enucleation) and radiotherapy. When both eyes are involved, the surgeon and patient may opt to remove the eye on the more severely affected side, and treat the opposite side with radiotherapy and/or chemotherapy in order to preserve vision.

CHAPTER 6. NEUROOPHTHALMOLOGY

Destruction of a cerebral hemisphere results in dense paralysis and sensory loss in the contralateral extremities. Such lesions do not result in corresponding visual loss or ocular paralysis confined to the contralateral eye. Rather, both eyes are affected partially. Neither eye can move to the side contralateral to the lesion and neither eye sees the contralateral environment (fig. 24).

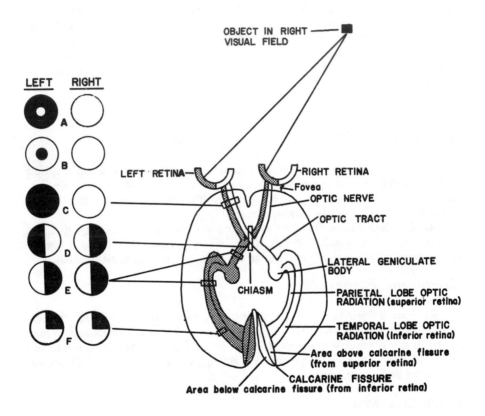

Figure 24. The visual pathways as seen from above the brain. Letters A-F refer to visual field defects following lesions in the corresponding brain areas. Circles indicate what the left and right eyes see (the left and right visual fields). Black areas represent visual field defects. A. Constricted field left eye (e.g., end-stage glaucoma). When constricted fields are bilateral, it sometimes signifies hysteria. B. Central scotoma (e.g., optic neuritis in multiple sclerosis). C. Total blindness of the left eye. D. Bitemporal hemianopia (e.g., pituitary gland tumor). E. Right homonymous hemianopia (e.g., stroke). F. Right superior quadrantopia. (From *Clinical Neuroanatomy Made Ridiculously Simple,* by S. Goldberg, MedMaster, 1979).

Optic fibers temporal to the fovea connect with the brain ipsilaterally. Fibers nasal to the fovea cross over to the opposite side at the optic chiasm. A lesion of the optic tract on the left, therefore, results in loss of the right visual field in each eye.

Note (fig. 24) that the right visual field falls on the left half of each retina; the superior visual field falls on the inferior retina. The right visual field projects to the left side of the brain. Similarly, the superior visual field projects below the calcarine fissure in the occipital lobe. In other words everything is upside down and backwards, provided you think in terms of visual fields. For example, a patient with a lesion below the right calcarine fissure experiences a left superior field defect (fig. 25)

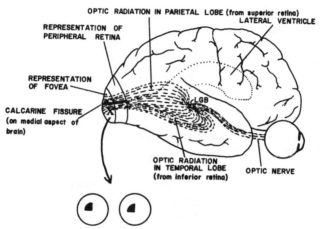

Figure 25. Lateral view of the visual pathways, showing the visual field defect resulting from a lesion (X) below the right calcarine fissure in the foveal region of the occipital cortex. LGB, lateral geniculate body. (Modified from Cushing, H., Trans. A. Neurol. Assoc., 47: 374-433, 1921).

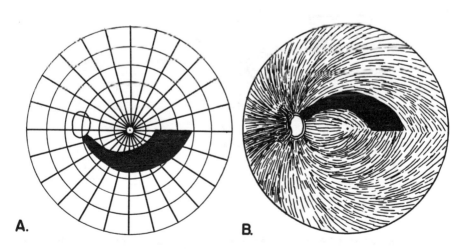

Figure 26. A. Visual field defect in early glaucoma. B. Corresponding damaged retinal area. It may be very difficult to detect the visual field defect without special equipment, like a tangent screen, or Goldmann perimeter.

The center of the retina (the fovea, which is the area of most acute vision) projects to the tip of the occipital lobe (fig. 25). Thus, a patient with a severe blow to the back of the head may experience bilateral central scotomas (visual field defects) if both occipital poles are destroyed. This fortunately is extremely rare.

OPTIC REFLEXES

Pupillary constriction to light

Unlike the pathways mediating vision, which involve a synapse in the lateral geniculate body, the pupillary light reflex involves a direct pathway to the midbrain from the optic tract (fig. 27). Shining a light in one eye normally leads to constriction of both pupils (termed the consensual reflex) as may be deduced from the connections depicted in figure 27. In severe optic nerve disease there will be no pupillary response when light is shined in the affected eye. There will be a consensual response when light is shined in the normal eye.

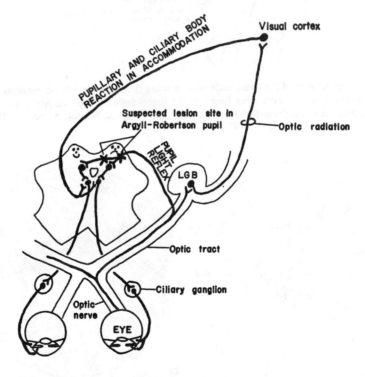

Figure 27. The pathways for the pupillary light reflex and accommodation. LGB, lateral geniculate body. The depicted lesions presumably also interrupt light reflex fibers crossing from the opposite side of the brain stem. The pathway shown innervating the eye is highly schematic; the light reflex pathway involves only pupillary constriction, whereas the accommodation pathway affects both pupillary constriction and ciliary body accommodation.

40

Accommodation

Accommodation (fig. 27) involves a neural circuit to the visual cortex and back, which makes sense, for we need our cerebral cortex to determine that something is out of focus before we can send directions to correct the focus. Focusing occurs by stimulating the smooth muscle of the ciliary body in the eye to contract, thereby enabling the lens to change its shape (accommodation). During accommodation not only does the lens focus but the pupil constricts, both smooth muscle actions mediated by parasympathetic components of CN3.

The syphilitic (Argyll-Robertson) pupil (also called the prostitute's pupil because it accommodates but does not react) constricts during accommodation, which is normal, but does not constrict to light. The lesion is considered to lie in the pretectal area of the superior colliculus (fig. 27). The condition is usually bilateral. The pupils characteristically are small and somewhat irregular (fig. 72E).

Conjugate gaze

Damage to the motor areas of the cerebral cortex produces contralateral paralysis of the extremities. It does not produce loss of all the contralateral eye muscle movements, but rather inpaired ability of either eye to look voluntarily toward the contralateral environment. Following a lesion to the left visuomotor area of the cerebrum, the patient cannot look to the right. His eyes tend to deviate to the left. In essence, they "look at the lesion". This occurs because the pathway from the left hemisphere innervates the right lateral rectus muscle (right CN6) and the left medial rectus muscle (left CN3). See figure 28. The right lateral rectus and left medial rectus muscles both direct the eyes to the right.

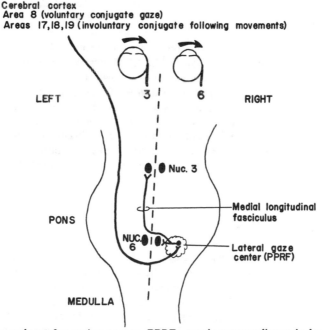

Figure 28. The pathway for conjugate gaze. PPRF - pontine paramedian reticular formation.

A bilateral lesion of the medial longitudinal fasciculus, most commonly seen in multiple sclerosis, would produce a decreased ability for either eye to look medially (figs. 28, 29). In this instance, both eyes could converge because the pathway for convergence (as well as vertical gaze) is different from the path for conjugate gaze. The condition resulting from lesions to the MLF is known as the *MLF (medial longitudinal fasciculus) syndrome* or *internuclear ophthalmoplegia* (fig. 29).

RIGHT   **LEFT**

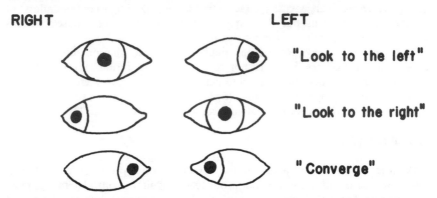

"Look to the left"

"Look to the right"

"Converge"

Figure 29. Internuclear ophthalmoplegia.

Convergence and vertical gaze apparently involve circuits in the midbrain close to (although not within) the superior colliculus. Hence, difficulty with convergence and vertical gaze may arise in tumors of the pineal gland which press upon the brain stem at the superior collicular level. *Parinaud's syndrome* is paralysis of vertical gaze following lesions close to the superior colliculus.

Nystagmus

Nystagmus is a repetitive involuntary, rhythmic tremor-like oscillating movement of the eyes. The most common form of nystagmus is horizontal jerk nystagmus, wherein the eyes repetitively move slowly toward one side and then quickly back. It is normal to have a slight degree of such nystagmus on attempting extreme lateral gaze, but marked degrees are abnormal and found in a variety of clinical conditions affecting the vestibular apparatus or brain stem. Vertical nystagmus is always abnormal, signifying a disorder in brain stem function. Pendular nystagmus, in which the eye moves at equal speeds in both directions, commonly is congenital or occurs after prolonged periods of bilateral blindness that begins in childhood.

Cranial nerve 7 (CN7)

CN7, the facial nerve, closes the eye via the orbicularis muscle, whereas CN3, the oculomotor nerve, opens the eye via the levator palpebrae muscle (fig. 10). In *Bell's palsy,* the facial nerve is compromised, resulting in total hemifacial paralysis, including difficulty with smiling, forehead wrinkling, and lid closure. In severe cases this results in drying of the eye, unless the lids are sutured together for the course of the disease, or lubricating medication is applied topically. The cause of the nerve injury is unclear. The usual site of injury in Bell's palsy is somewhere in the facial canal (which lies between the internal acoustic meatus and the stylomastoid foramen - fig. 30), and may involve other branches of CN7 (to the stapedius muscle, lacrimal and salivary glands (fig. 30). Since the stapedius dampens sound waves, its nonfunctioning leads to hyperacusis, wherein sounds appear excessively loud. Bell's palsy usually improves spontaneously within 4-6 weeks. The patient may then, however, experience "crocodile tears", in which the patient tears on eating, instead of salivating. This results from misguided growth of the regenerating salivary and lacrimal axons.

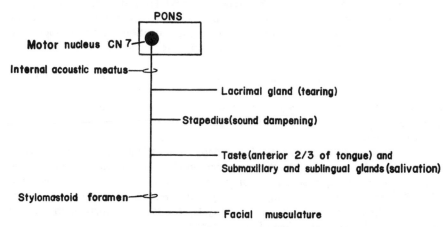

Figure 30. Schematic view of the course of cranial nerve 7.

When the cerebral cortex is injured on one side, facial weakness is manifest below the opposite eye, with little disability of eyelid closure or eyebrow elevation. This sparing of the upper face occurs because *each* cerebral hemisphere normally innervates the entire forehead and both eyelids. When one hemisphere is damaged, the other carries on the function.

Cranial Nerve 5 (CN5)

CN5, the trigeminal nerve, transmits sensation from the eye, particularly touch and pain from the cornea. It is important in the blink reflex to corneal touch. Damage to the nerve may result in corneal erosions, in part due to corneal exposure and drying. Herpes zoster, a disease of peripheral nerves, may affect the trigeminal nerve. When the ophthalmic division of CN5 is affected, the patient develops a typical herpetic vesicular rash that affects the eyelids and forehead to the midline. Uveitis may develop, and an ophthalmologist should see the patient if the eye appears to be affected. Therapy may include pain medication, dilating drops, and topical and/or systemic steroids.

Migraine and temporal arteritis

Classic *migraine* is a throbbing, commonly unilateral headache, associated with nausea, and preceded by a prodrome (e.g., visual disturbances, hemiparesis, dizziness). The visual aura are particularly common and may consist of wave-like rippling or other defects in the visual field, whether uniocular or binocular. Migraine

43

commonly is familial. The aura phase is believed due to vasoconstriction, which is followed by a phase of vasodilation and arterial wall edema (the headache phase). The condition must be distinguished from transient ischemic attacks, neurological deficits which are believed due to microemboli and in which the nausea and headache are not prominent features. Also, transient ischemic attacks tend to be briefer (lasting a few seconds or minutes). Occasionally, a migraine attack will result in a permanent neurologic deficit.

Migraine treatment may include analgesics, sedatives, antidepressants, biofeedback, periactin, propranolol (a beta-adrenergic blocker) or more specific medication - the ergot derivatives or, for prophylaxis, methysergide (Sansert). As the ergot derivatives are vasoconstrictors they must be used with caution when neurologic aura are pronounced, as these agents, while helping the headache, may worsen the neurologic deficit.

Cluster headache is a variant of migraine. The patient experiences headaches in clusters - several times daily over several weeks, followed by weeks or months of remission. The eye becomes red and the headache may be excruciating. It commonly is worse at night and exacerbated by alcohol ingestion. The treatment is similar to that of migraine.

Temporal arteritis is a disease of the elderly. The patient typically experiences a unilateral headache centering around the temporal artery, which is tender to the touch. The erythrocyte sedimentation rate is markedly elevated (greater than 50mm/hr) and biopsy of the temporal artery may reveal an inflammatory reaction. Attacks of blindness are common, and may be due to thrombosis of the central retinal artery. Steroids are often of great benefit.

CHAPTER 7. OCULAR FINDINGS IN SYSTEMIC DISEASE

AIDS: Retinopathy with "cotton wool" spots on retina; Kaposi's sarcoma of eyelids and conjunctiva; keratitis; herpes zoster; uveitis; candida chorioretinitis.

ALBINISM: Light fundus background (choroidal vessels seen easily with the ophthalmoscope as pigment epithelium is unpigmented; nystagmus; poor vision (high refractive errors and poor macular development); pink-blue iris (iris transilluminates).

ALKAPTONURIA: Melanin deposits in sclera (at 9 and 3 o'clock positions around the cornea).

AMYLOIDOSIS: Weakness of extraocular muscles; vitreous opacities; pupillary abnormalities; amyloid nodules in lids and conjunctiva.

ANEMIA: Conjunctiva appears pale; retinal hemorrhages and exudates.

ANKYLOSING SPONDYLITIS: Uveitis; scleritis; scleromalacia perforans (thinning of sclera with exposure of uveal tissue).

ATOPIC DERMATITIS: Cataracts; keratoconus.

BEHCET'S SYNDROME: Uveitis.

CYSTIC FIBROSIS: Papilledema; retinal hemorrhages.

CYSTINOSIS: Deposits of cystine crystals in cornea and conjunctiva.

CYTOMEGALIC INCLUSION DISEASE (congenital): Chorioretinitis, cataracts.

DERMATOMYOSITIS: Extraocular muscle palsies; lid edema; scleritis; uveitis, retinal exudates.

DIABETES MELLITUS: Extraocular muscle palsies; Xanthelasmae; retinal microaneurysms; hemorrhages, exudates and neovascularization of the retina; cataracts; rubeosis iridis (neovascularization of the iris); glaucoma.

DOWN'S SYNDROME: Up-and-out obliquity to the lids; Brushfield's spots (white speckling of iris); cataracts; myopia; strabismus.

EHLERS-DANLOS SYNDROME: Blue sclera; strabismus; epicanthal folds.

FREIDRICH'S ATAXIA: Nystagmus; strabismus; retinitis pigmentosa.

GALACTOSEMIA: Cataracts.

GLOMERULONEPHRITIS: Periorbital edema; Hypertensive retinopathy.

GOUT: Episcleritis, uveitis; deposition of uric acid crystals in cornea.

HEREDITARY HEMORRHAGIC TELANGIECTASIA (Osler-Weber-Rendu disease): Telangiectasias of conjunctiva and retina.

HERPES ZOSTER: Dermatitis along ophthalmic branch of cranial nerve 5; uveitis; keratitis.

HISTOPLASMOSIS: Chorioretinal scars, retinal hemorrhage.

HOMOCYSTINURIA: Dislocated lens.

HYPERLIPIDEMIA: Xanthelasmae, arcus juvenilis, lipemia retinalis (milky retinal vessels secondary to excessive lipids in the blood).

HYPERPARATHYROIDISM: Band keratopathy (grey-white band, containing calcium deposits, extending horizontally across the cornea); optic atrophy.

HYPERTHYROIDISM: Proptosis, lid retraction; infrequent blinking (staring); lid lag on downward gaze; weakness of upward gaze; poor convergence; diplopia; corneal erosions (from poor lid closure); papilledema; papillitis (fig. 57).

HYPOPARATHYROIDISM: Cataracts; papilledema; optic neuritis.

HYPOTHROIDISM (Congenital cretinism): Strabismus; farsightedness; cataracts; swollen lids with narrow slits between lids; wide set eyes; retrobulbar neuritis; optic atrophy; loss of outer half of eyebrows.

IMPENDING STROKE: Amaurosis fugax (transient blindness from intermittent vascular compromise in arteriosclerotic disease); Hollenhorst plaques (glistening emboli seen at branch points of retinal arterioles).

KERNICTERUS (erythroblastosis fetalis): Strabismus; nystagmus; retinal hemorrhage.

LEAD POISONING: Papilledema; optic atrophy.

LUPUS ERYTHEMATOSIS: Retinal hemorrhages; cotton wool exudates; papilledema; lid lesions similar to lesions elsewhere; episcleritis; keratitis; uveitis; nystagmus; extraocular muscle palsies; cataracts.

MACROGLOBULINEMIA: Venous occlusion (engorged retinal veins with hemorrhages and exudates); papilledema.

MARCHESANI'S SYNDROME: Dislocated lens.

MARFAN'S SYNDROME: Dislocated lens.

MIGRAINE: Throbbing eye pain; transient visual compromise (e.g., flashing lights, waves, hemianopia); miotic (small) pupil (sympathetic axon compromise with carotid artery wall edema).

MUCOPOLYSACCHARIDOSES: Corneal clouding.

MULTIPLE SCLEROSIS: Retrobulbar neuritis; optic atrophy; internuclear ophthalmoplegia; strabismus.

MYASTHENIA GRAVIS: Ptosis; extraocular muscle paresis.

MYOTONIA: Cataracts.

NEUROFIBROMATOSIS: Lid and orbital tumors; optic gliomas.

OSTEOGENESIS IMPERFECTA: Blue sclera (choroid shows through thin sclera).

POLYARTERITIS NODOSA: Episcleritis; corneal ulcers, uveitis; retinal hemorrhages and exudates; papilledema; hypertensive retinopathy; arteriolar occlusion.

POLYCYTHEMIA: Markedly dilated retinal veins; papilledema.

PSEUDOXANTHOMA ELASTICUM: Angioid streaks (reddish bands radiating from disc region, resembling blood vessels; probably represent defects in the choroidal membrane (Bruch's membrane) just outside the pigment epithelium. Also found in Paget's disease of the bone and sickle cell disease).

RADIATION EXPOSURE: Cataracts; retinopathy.

REITER'S SYNDROME: Uveitis; retinal vasculitis.

RHEUMATOID ARTHRITIS: Uveitis; band keratopathy; scleromalacia perforans (degeneration and thinning of anterior sclera with bulging out of underlying bluish choroid).

RILEY-DAY SYNDROME (familial dysautonomia): Decreased tear production; decreased corneal sensation with subsequent exposure keratitis.

ROSACEA: Blepharitis; conjunctivitis; keratitis; episcleritis.

RUBELLA (congenital): Cataracts; microphthalmia; cloudy corneas; uveitis; pigmentary retinopathy.

SARCOID: Uveitis; whitish perivenous infiltrates in retina (fig. 70); band keratopathy.

SICKLE CELL ANEMIA: Retinal hemorrhages, exudates, microaneurysms, neovascularization (vascular and hemorrhagic changes are worse in the sickle C than in sickle S disease); papilledema; angioid streaks.

SJOGREN'S SYNDROME: Dry eyes; corneal erosions.

STEVENS-JOHNSON SYNDROME: Purulent conjunctivitis with scarring of conjunctiva and cornea.

SUBACUTE BACTERIAL ENDOCARDITIS: Conjunctival and retinal hemorrhages; Roth spots (retinal hemorrhages with white centers - fig. 62).

STURGE-WEBER DISEASE: Congenital glaucoma on side of facial nevus.

SYPHILIS: Interstitial keratitis (inflammation, edema, and vascular infiltration of the cornea, particularly the corneal periphery); uveitis; optic neuritis; cataracts; chorioretinitis; lens dislocation; Argyll-Robertson pupil (fig. 72E).

TAY-SACHS DISEASE: Cherry red spot (cloudiness of retina, except in fovea region).

TEMPORAL ARTERITIS: Transient or permanent loss of vision from vasculitis affecting the optic nerve.

TOXEMIA: Hypertensive retinopathy.

TOXOPLASMOSIS: Chorioretinitis.

TRICHINOSIS: Inflammation of extraocular muscles.

TUBERCULOSIS: Uveitis; chorioretinitis.

TUBEROUS SCLEROSIS: Retinal tumors.

ULCERATIVE COLITIS: Uveitis.

VITAMIN DEFICIENCIES:
   Vitamin A deficiency - Night blindness; xerophthalmia (drying of cornea and conjunctiva).
   Thiamine deficiency (beriberi) - Optic neuritis; extraocular muscle weakness.
   Niacin deficiency (pellagra) - Optic neuritis.
   Riboflavin deficiency - Photophobia; inflammation of conjunctiva and cornea.
   Vitamin C deficiency (scurvy) - Hemorrhages within and outside the eye.
   Vitamin D deficiency - Cataracts; papilledema (as in hypoparathyroidism).

VON HIPPEL-LINDAU DISEASE: Retinal hemangiomas.

WILM'S TUMOR: Aniridia (absence of iris).

WILSON'S DISEASE: Copper deposits in Descement's membrane in the peripheral cornea (Kayser-Fleischer ring) and in the lens (copper cataracts).

DRUG EFFECTS

CHLORAMPHENICOL: Optic neuritis.

CHLOROQUINE: Drug deposits in cornea and lens; pigmentary retinopathy.

CHLORPROMAZINE (Thorazine): Deposits in cornea and lens; pigmentary retinopathy; blurred vision.

CONTRACEPTIVE HORMONES: Decreased corneal tolerance to contact lenses; migraine; optic neuritis; central vein occlusion.

DIGITALIS: Yellow vision.

DIURETICS: Myopia.

ETHAMBUTOL: Retrobulbar neuritis with decreased color vision and visual acuity.

GOLD: Gold keratitis.

HALOPERIDOL (Haldol): Oculogyric crises; blurred vision.

THIORIDAZINE (Mellaril): Pigmentary retinopathy.

STEROIDS: Cataracts and glaucoma (from topical or systemic steroids); papilledema (from systemic steroids).

TETRACYCLINE: Papilledema.

VITAMIN A INTOXICATION: Papilledema.

VITAMIN D INTOXICATION: Band keratopathy.

CHAPTER 8. OPHTHALMOLOGIC TECHNIQUES

A. Assessment of Visual Acuity

   The first part of any eye exam should be visual acuity testing. This is both for diagnostic purposes, as well as for legal reasons (the patient may gain the impression that vision declined after you touched the eye). The most common tests for visual acuity are the distance (Snellen) vision chart and near (Rosenbaum) vision chart. For illiterate patients, charts with numbers rather than letters may be more suitable. Many people who do not know the letters do know numbers. For small children, charts with pictures, or the "E" symbol arranged in different positions, may be more suitable.

   Test one eye at a time! When covering either eye, be sure the patient does not press on the eye, as this may transiently interfere with visual acuity. Examples of terminology: 20/100 means the patient at 20 feet can read no more lines than a normal person can read at 100 feet. 20/30 + 2 means the patient read the 20/30 line plus 2 letters on the 20/25 line. 20/30 − means the patient read the 20/30 line except for 2 letters. 20/200 with best correction is considered legally blind. Vision may be recorded up to 20/400 or 20/800 but beyond that is recorded as FC (Finger-counting), HM (Hand Motion), LP (Light Perception), and NLP (No Light Perception). Test the patient with his glasses. Be sure to check, however, whether the glasses are for distance, for near, or for both (bifocals). Use the distance glasses for testing distance and near (reading) glasses for near vision.

B. The Direct Ophthalmoscope

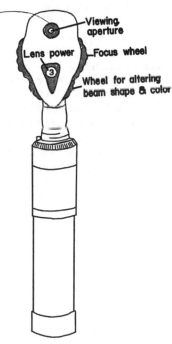

Figure 31. The direct ophthalmoscope.

This commonly employed instrument, used both by ophthalmologists and non-ophthalmologists, is pictured in figure 31. Note the two main wheels - one for focusing the lens and one for changing the shape or color of the light beam. The black numbers on the focus wheel represent spherical convex (positive) lenses. These lenses converge light rays. The red numbers are spherical concave (negative) lenses. These lenses diverge light rays. The ophthalmoscope does not contain cylindrical lenses. Lenses are necessary because different people have different refractive errors, and the appropriate lens is necessary to focus on the retina. Most of the beam shapes are seldom employed by ophthalmologists, as they are not especially helpful. Most helpful are the large and small circular white beams. The larger round beam is used most frequently and provides the broadest view of the fundus. The smaller white round beam is used when the pupil is small, and there is too much glare from light that backscatters from the iris.

How to examine the patient

1. Use your right eye to visualize the right eye and your left eye to visualize the left eye. Otherwise a potentially embarassing social situation may develop, and you will need a supply of breath mints. If you have but one good eye, then it is permissible to view the patient head on, although it is still not necessary. The patient could lie down while you examine from a position behind the patient's head.

2. Have the patient look at a distant object. If the patient instead looks right into your light, all you will ever see is the fovea, which is following and focusing on your light.

3. Obtain a red reflex (the pupil appears red) in the patient's eye while looking through the ophthalmoscope. (When the ophthalmoscope is not used, the pupil normally appears black).

4. Move close to the patient, close enough to rest your hand on the patient's cheek. Use the large round white light, unless there is too much glare, in which case the small round white light should be used.

5. Starting with focusing wheel on O, move the wheel back and forth until a setting is found with a segment of retinal vessel in focus. The proper etiquette is to use the index finger on the focusing wheel.

6. Follow the retinal vessel back to the optic disc. Do not be dismayed if your field of view is very narrow, not at all panoramic as in the textbook pictures. No one can see much more than one disc diameter with the visual field of a direct ophthalmoscope. It is necessary to tilt the instrument to different positions to piece together the composite picture of the fundus.

7. The optic disc lies slightly nasal to the center of the retina. Examine the optic disc from *out to in,* first noting the disc margin. Is it well-outlined (normal), or blurred (as in papilledema)? Then note the color of the disc. Is it normal pink-white, or white, as in optic atrophy? Or is it angry-looking with dilated tortuous vessels, as in papilledema? Note the cup size. Is there a normal cup/disc diameter ratio of about ⅓ or is the cup small or large? Actually the cup may normally be small or large, but it is abnormal for it to be large in one eye and small in the other. Normally, cups are about the same size in each eye. Glaucoma causes a large scooped-out cup (fig. 22). In papilledema, the cup is small or absent.

8.   Examine the blood vessels that enter the cup. Is there venous pulsation in the region of the disc where the veins enter the cup? You should be able to see venous pulsation in most eyes. If venous pulsation is present, it strongly suggests that there is no papilledema, because venous pulsation is one of the first things to disappear with papilledema. The absence of venous pulsation does not tell you much, since it may be difficult to detect in normals.

9.   Follow out as far as you can (generally just beyond the fovea) the four arcades of blood vessels, each a paired arteriole and vein. There is considerable variation in this patterning. Are there hemorrhages or exudates (which may be found in ateriolar or venous disease or in blood dyscrasias); narrowed tortuous arterioles, as may be found in hypertension and other conditions? Normally the veins have a larger diameter than the arterioles in a ratio of about 5/3. Do the arterioles have a normal light reflex or is the reflex broadened, as is found in chronic hypertension (fig. 23)? Is the blood column clearly seen in the arterioles or is there copper or silver wiring, a sign of thickening of the arteriolar media, found in chronic hypertension? Are there retinal lesions (figs. 60-70)?

10.   Examine the fovea, which lies about 2 disc diameters temporal to the optic disc. In young individuals it is seen as a pinpoint light reflection. In older individuals, one may only see a general area of increased pigmentation. Note any *intense* pigmentation, distortions or hemorrhages that may signify macular degeneration. One may also find the fovea by asking the patient to look into the light. This, however, induces increased pupillary constriction and the excess glare may inhibit visualization.

Dilating drops may be used if it is difficult to visualize the retina. Don't use atropine; it will paralyze accommodation (cause *cycloplegia)* for two weeks. Don't use cyclopentolate (Cyclogyl). It may paralyze accommodation for 1 day. The latter agents are used in situations where one wants either prolonged pupillary dilation (as in uveitis) or a strong cycloplegia (as in uveitis or in performing a cycloplegic refraction). Rather, use a short acting dilator like tropicamide (Mydriacil) 0.5-1.0% which lasts only 6 hrs. Mydriacil is a parasympathetic inhibitor. Hence, it not only dilates the pupil but paralyzes accommodation. If you wish only to dilate the pupil, use phenylephrine (Neosynephrine) 2.5-10%. It is a sympathomimetic agent; it causes pupillary dilation but does not affect accommodation because the ciliary body does not have a significant sympathetic innervation. Both Mydriacil and Neosynephrine take effect in about 20-30 minutes and last about 6 hours. One or two drops applied once should suffice. The best pupillary dilation is obtained by using Mydriacil and Neosynephrine simultaneously.

Since about 2% of the population over 40 will develop glaucoma and about 5% of these are of the angle closure type (one out of 1,000 patients), it is unlikely that you will induce an attack of angle closure by using dilating drops. Even if you do, the symptoms are readily apparent and easily treated (see Chapter 3). Do not, however, use dilating drops on neurological patients for whom a change in pupillary diameter may be an important sign. Don't use them in patients with known angle closure glaucoma or in patients who have had an artificial lens implant - the lens may then fall into the vitreous chamber. If you are still nervous administering drops, note that only patients with shallow anterior chamber angles can have an attack of angle closure. A simple method of assessing the depth of the angle is described in Section F.

C. The Indirect Ophthalmoscope

In indirect ophthalmoscopy, the examiner wears a bright headlight for direct illumination and examines the retina through a hand-held lens (fig. 32). This technique has the advantage over direct ophthalmoscopy in that the observer can visualize the retina through moderate cataracts, and also can see a much wider field than with the direct ophthalmoscope. With special manipulations, one can even view the retinal periphery. The disadvantage of the technique is that everything appears smaller than with the direct ophthalmoscope and also upside down, making this a much more difficult technique to master than direct ophthalmoscopy. In general, indirect ophthalmoscopy is used only by ophthalmologists.

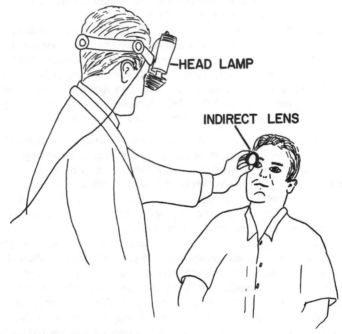

Figure 32. The indirect ophthalmoscope.

D. The Application of Fluorescein Strips and Ophthalmic Drops and Ointments

Fluorescein formerly was supplied as drops, but when pseudomonas was found growing in a number of the bottles, paper strips superceded. It is necessary to get only a small amount of fluorescein into the eye for satisfactory viewing. If the eye is tearing, it is unnecessary to wet the strip. If the eye is dry, it is necessary to wet only one corner of the strip with water or saline. Do not touch the cornea, as this is painful. Touch the lower fornix with the strip while the patient looks up. A blue or fluorescent light will illuminate the fluorescein, which will collect in corneal areas having a break in the surface epithelium.

Ophthalmic drops as well as ointments should similarly be applied to the lower fornix so as to avoid irritating the cornea. As the eye only holds one or two drops, there is little concern about applying too much. The excess will not stay in the eye. The abbreviation "gtt" on a prescription refers to "drops".

In the not-uncommon patient who panics and blinks his lids spasmodically on attempting to apply drops, a simple technique suffices. Have the patient lie supine, with the eyes closed. Place the drops on the skin in the pocket between the nose and nasal aspect of the lids. Then, have the patient open his eyes; the drops will enter the eye.

E.   The Schiotz Tonometer

The patient should lie flat, with eyes looking up at the ceiling. Place 1-2 drops of topical ocular anesthetic in the eye. Gently part the eyelids being very careful not to press on the eye. Pressure on the eye will raise intraocular pressure artifactually. Rest the base of the tonometer on the cornea with the instrument maintained in a vertical position. In virtually all cases, the 5.5 gram weight will suffice (figs. 33, 34). For the most accuracy, use sufficient weight to obtain a scale reading of at least "four". Move the barrel of the shaft half way down to the base of the instrument. Record the scale number and read the corresponding pressure on the accompanying Schiotz chart. A pressure of over 21 mm is grounds for referral to an ophthalmologist for visual field testing. Many ophthalmologists will not treat an elevated pressure, unless there is some sign of beginning field loss, as certain patients may have high pressure and never suffer damage. Treatment with glaucoma drops is a lifelong commitment.

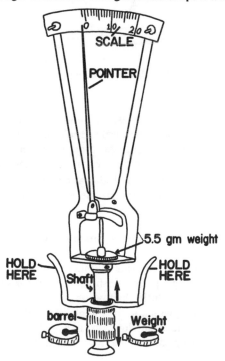

Figure 33. The Schiotz tonometer. The barrel can move up or down (arrows) along the shaft.

The correct barrel position is midway along the shaft, when reading the patient's pressure. The 5.5 gram weight is permanently affixed to the tonometer. Additional weights may be added to this, to obtain a scale reading of at least "four".

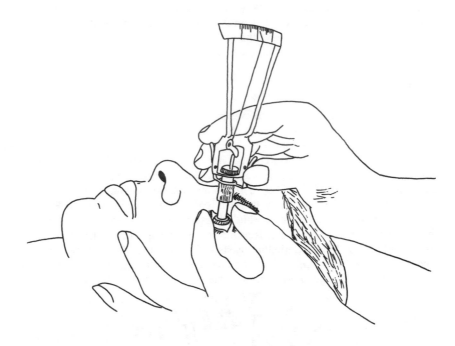

Figure 34. Correct positioning of the Schiotz tonometer.

Calibrate the tonometer before use by applying it to the accompanying small round metal platform. The tonometer scale should read "O", which translates to a very high pressure - "rock hard" on the tonometer chart. Wipe the base of the tonometer with alcohol before and after use for sterility and to prevent dirt from accumulating, which might throw off the calibration. Be sure to allow the alcohol to dry off before placing the tonometer on the eye, or the alcohol may "fix" the epithelial cells.

F.   Assessing the Depth of the Anterior Chamber Angle

A simple assessment of the anterior chamber depth and narrowness of the angle may be performed by shining a pocket flashlight onto the iris from the side (fig. 35). In the normal patient there is little shadow on the iris on the opposite side of the pupil. In a shallow chamber, with a narrow angle (fig. 35C, D), the iris is bowed forward. Thus, there is a significant shadow, just as a light shined from one side of a hill results in a shadow on the opposite slope. Practice this technique to become familiar with the normal.

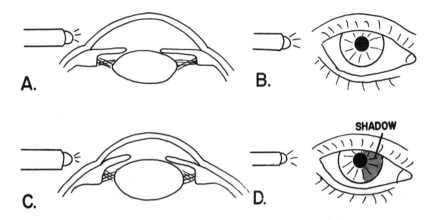

Figure 35. Assessing the depth of the anterior chamber. A and B, normal. C and D. Shallow chamber with narrow angle. A shadow forms because of the oblique positioning of the iris.

The ophthalmologist uses a more sophisticated instrument to examine the angle, a goniolens. This is modified contact lens with mirrors that can be used with the slit lamp to peer into the angle of the anterior chamber and also to view the retinal periphery and other retinal areas.

G.   Removal of a Foreign Body

Application of anesthetic drops may facilitate the examination of the eye for a foreign body. Both proparacaine (Ophthaine) and tetracaine (Pontocaine) drops take effect within a few seconds and last about 10-25 minutes.

Check the lid margin. Are any lashes pointing inward and rubbing against the eye? Sometimes the lid margin is turned inward, termed *entropion* (as opposed to *ectropion,* where the lid is turned outward, exposing the conjunctival surface of the lid to the air, with subsequent irritation - see figs. 42, 43). Is an eyelash trapped in the lacrimal punctum? - a simple thing to remove with tweezers. Have the patient look in all directions, to detect a foreign body on the globe. Pull down the lower lid to check on the conjunctival surface. With the patient looking down, grasp the upper-lid margin at the base of the lashes; then evert the upper lid (fig. 36) to check for any foreign body - often a miniscule particle of dirt trapped in the lid and easily removed with a cotton applicator. Fluorescein will enhance visualization of a foreign body on the cornea. Vertical scratch marks on the cornea suggest a foreign body under the upper eyelid, which abrades the cornea with each blink.

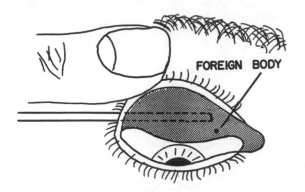

Figure 36. Technique of inverting the upper lid. Grasp the upper lid and lashes at the eyelash margin and flip the lid back over a wooden applicator stick or pencil.

If you find a foreign body embedded in the cornea, try irrigating it out (after applying topical anesthetic drops) with a stream of water or saline from a syringe or ocular irrigation bottle. If unsuccessful, the foreign body may lie deep in the cornea (remember the cornea is only about 1 mm thick), and it is advisable to refer the patient to an ophthalmologist who will remove the foreign body under a slit lamp.

H. Securing an Eye Patch

In securing an eye patch, place one end of the tape near the center of the forehead. Otherwise the other end will lie awkwardly on the nose. Place the other end on the cheek bone, not near the mouth, where chewing and talking movements will continually move the patch (fig. 37).

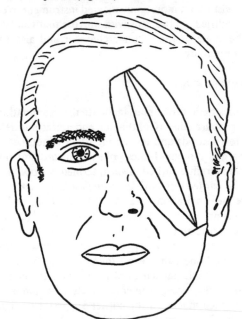

Figure 37. Correct position for an eyepatch.

I. The Slit Lamp (Fig. 37A)

The slit lamp will not be discussed in detail except to point out its usefulness. It magnifies. One also can alter the shape of the light beam to facilitate viewing in certain unique ways. A slit-like beam facilitates visualization of the layers of the cornea and lens; one can thus evaluate the thickness of these structures and more accurately localize disease processes. A pinpoint beam facilitates the examination of the anterior chamber for the Tyndall effect - a subtle sign of intraocular hemorrhage or inflammation. Most slit lamps also have a sensitive tonometer for accurate recording of intraocular pressure.

J. Cataract Surgery

Cataract extraction is usually an elective procedure, except when the lens is *hypermature* (requires a slit lamp to determine this). A hypermature lens is densely opaque, swollen, and leaky. This may result in glaucoma or uveitis if the lens is not extracted. Most surgeons consider a visual acuity of 20/70 or worse (from cataracts) as grounds for cataract extraction. Each case must be individualized, however. A watchmaker with 20/40 vision may require cataract extaction to perform his job well. An elderly, illiterate person may get along quite well with 20/200 vision.

The ophthalmoscope provides a good clue as to whether visual loss is due to cataracts or to other intraocular disease (e.g. macular degeneration). "If the examiner can see in, the patient can see out." I.e., if the examiner can see the retina clearly using the ophthalmoscope it is unlikely that the cataract is sufficiently dense to cause a significant problem in visual acuity (see also fig. 72F). Judgment is necessary to determine whether or not to remove a uniocular cataract (see pg. 20).

Most ophthalmologists perform cataract surgery under local anesthesia, although general anesthesia may also be used. Two injections are generally used for local nerve blocks. The facial nerve is blocked, as eyelid blinking during the time of surgery may cause the contents of the eye to extrude. Facial nerve block is performed either at the mandibular joint or just lateral to the eyelids. As eyeball movements must be eliminated, local anesthetic is also administered by injection behind the eye in the muscle cone of the extraocular muscles. The eye is then open via an incision at the periphery of the cornea (generally extending about 160° superiorly). A narrow freezing probe (cryoprobe) is introduced into the eye and freezes to the lens, which is then pulled out. The cornea is then sutured closed.

Some surgeons, instead of using a cryoprobe, use a narrow ultravibratory instrument (a *phacoemulsifier)* which breaks up the lens into small fragments that are suctioned out. This technique requires only a small corneal incision, as the lens is not removed as a whole. In order to avoid complications of the emulsification procedure, it is important that the surgeon be well-skilled in the technique, and that the instrument be applied only to the lens.

It is routine, during cataract surgery, to create one or more holes in the iris (iridectomy - see fig. 72A, B). This facilitates drainage of aqueous humor into the anterior chamber in the event that vitreous gel plugs the pupil.

Complications of cataract surgery include intraocular hemorrhage, infection, corneal opacification from corneal trauma, loss of vitreous (which fortunately can be replaced with saline), retinal detachment, wound leakage, and glaucoma (from plugging of the pupil with vitreous gel, and from collapse of the anterior chamber). The success rate is high, however, in view of excellent advances in surgical technique, including fine needles and sutures, and specially designed surgical instruments.

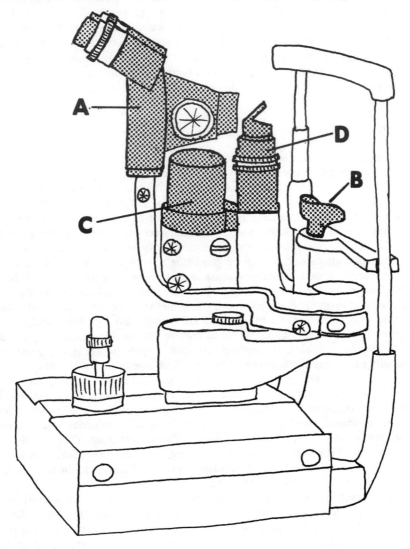

Figure 37A. The Slit Lamp. A, stereoscopic microscope; B, chin rest for patient; C, light source; D, adjustable slit mechanism.

CHAPTER 9. CLINICAL REVIEW

EYE SYMPTOMS *Visual Disturbances*	MOST COMMON DIAGNOSES
Acute spontaneous loss of vision in one eye, transient.	1. Transient ischemic attack involving blood circulation to retina. Lasting deficit may indicate central retinal artery occlusion or arteriolar or venous hemorrhage. 2. Migraine 3. Temporal arteritis
Acute spontaneous loss of vision in both eyes, transient.	1. Transient ischemic attack involving blood circulation to visual areas of brain. 2. Migraine
Floaters (particles of dust, spots, cobwebs). No other visual difficulties.	Vitreous opacities, usually insignificant.
Lightning flashes.	1. Migraine (often also manifest as "wavy" appearance to environment); 2. may accompany traction on retina or retinal detachment.
Curtain drawn over an eye.	Retinal detachment or hemorrhage.
Blurred vision - far only.	Myopia.
Blurred vision - near only.	Hyperopia; use of cyloplegic drops; presbyopia.
Double vision.	Nerve or muscle damage. If monocular, may reflect lens dislocation or cataract.
Vertigo (spinning of patient or environment).	Dysfunction of vestibular apparatus or its connection in the brain stem.
Loss of central vision in one eye.	Macular or optic nerve disease.

360° loss of peripheral vision in each eye (sparing of macular region).	Glaucoma; hysteria; certain drug toxicities(e.g., quinine, chloroquine); retinitis pigmentosa.
Loss of side (lateral) vision in both eyes.	Optic chiasm lesion.
Loss in both eyes of ability to perceive the right (or left) environment.	Lesion of optic tract or optic radiation.
Loss of night vision.	Retinitis pigmentosa; vitamin A deficiency.
Halos around lights.	Glaucoma (from corneal edema); cataracts.
Yellow vision.	Digitalis toxicity.
Ocular Discomfort Eye fatigue (asthenopia).	Hyperopia; prolonged near work; muscle imbalance.
Itching.	Allergy.
Acute onset superficial sticking pain.	Foreign body.
Burning.	Conjunctivitis; corneal irritation; eye strain; allergy; dry eyes.
Deep intense pain.	Uveitis; glaucoma; optic neuritis; referred vascular pain (e.g., aneurysm, migraine), sinusitis; tension headache.
Pain upon pressing on the globe.	Lid or orbital inflammation; scleritis and episcleritis; anterior uveitis; angle closure glaucoma.
Sensitivity to light (photophobia).	Conjunctivitis; keratitis (inflammation of cornea), uveitis.

| Headache centering in the eye. | Refractive error; inflammation of the eye or its surroundings; migraine; tension headache; sinusitis; angle closure glaucoma; uveitis; side effects of glaucoma medication; cerebral lesion. |

EYE SIGNS

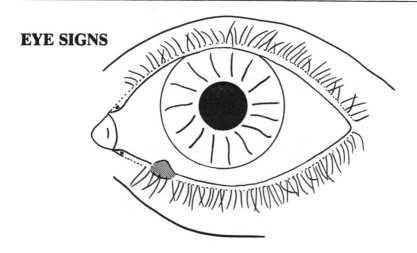

Figure 38. Tender, smooth, reddish pimple on lid margin, arising within the past week.

Diagnosis: Stye

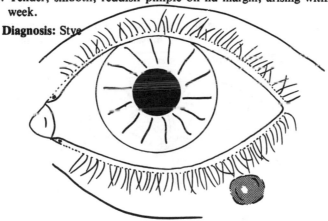

Figure 39. Minimally tender, smooth, well-outlined, firm bump, some distance from the lid margin.

Diagnosis: Chalazion

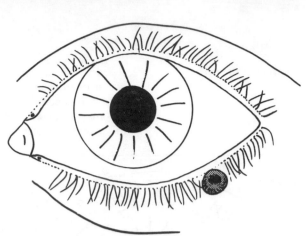

Figure 40. Dimpled, firm, pearly, ulcerated lesion on lower lid.

Diagnosis: Basal cell carcinoma.

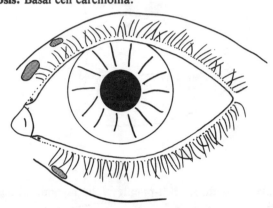

Figure 41. Soft, yellowish superficial skin lesions in a patient with hyperlipidemia. (Also commonly found in diabetics but may be found in normal individuals).

Diagnosis: Xanthelasmae

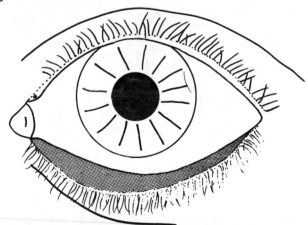

Figure 42. Conjunctival surface of lower lid red and exposed.

Diagnosis: Ectropion (eversion of lid).

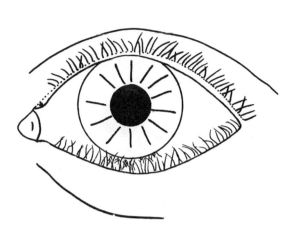

Figure 43. Foreign body sensation in eye.

Diagnosis: Entropion (inversion of lid).

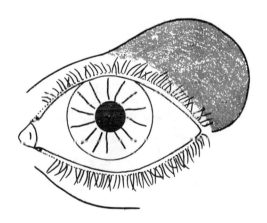

Figure 44. Warm, painful swelling, acutely arising, in superolateral aspect of upper lid.

Diagnosis: Dacryoadenitis (lacrimal gland inflammation); may be secondary to bacterial, spirochetal, viral, or fungal infections; treated with warm soaks and systemic antibiotics; may also result from tumors.

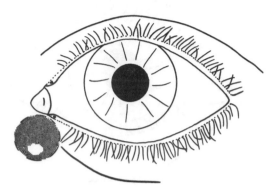

Figure 45. Warm, painful swelling, nasal aspect lower lid; drainage of pus back through lacrimal puncta.

Diagnosis: Dacryocystitis (inflammation of lacrimal sac); usually due to *staphylococcus aureus* but may also result from other bacteria, spirochetes, viruses, or fungi; treated with massage of the lacrimal sac, warm compresses and antibiotic ointments. Abscesses may require incision and drainage.

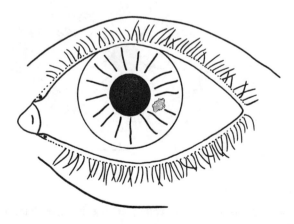

Figure 46. Painful foreign body sensation in eye scratched by a finger nail earlier in the day. Strong fluorescein uptake of an isolated area of cornea.

Diagnosis: Corneal abrasion. Treat with topical antibiotics and an eye patch until healed (usually within 1-2 days).

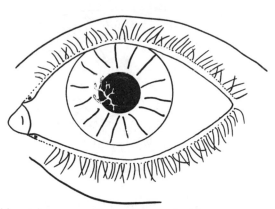

Figure 47. Photophobia, redness, sometimes decreased vision.

Diagnosis: Herpes simplex (dendritic ulcer). See page 24.

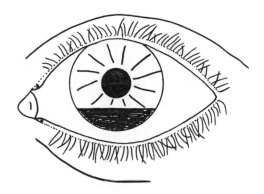

Figure 48. Blunt trauma to eye with decrease in vision.

Diagnosis: Hyphema; usually resolves spontaneously. Requires bed rest and bilateral patching to decrease eye movements.

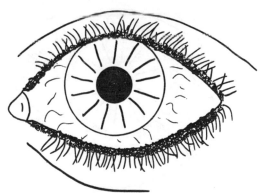

Figure 49. Crusty, mildly sore eyelids; eyelids stick together in the morning.

Diagnosis: Blepharitis (inflammation of eyelids). May be secondary to dandruff (seborrheic dermatitis) or infection (usually *staphylococcus aureus);* Rx: dandruff control, topical antibiotics.

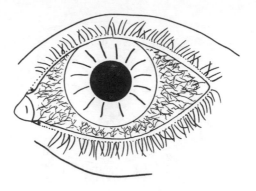

Figure 50. Mildly irritated red eye, no history of trauma; flu-like syndrome.

Diagnosis: Conjunctivitis, probably viral. A crusty eyelash margin makes a bacterial cause more likely.

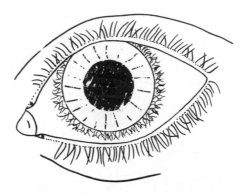

Figure 51. Entire eye is very painful; hazy vision; halos around lights.

Diagnosis: Acute (closed angle) glaucoma. Note vascular prominence around perimeter of cornea, mid-dilated pupil.

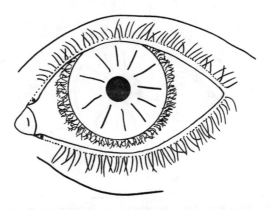

Figure 52. Marked photophobia, decreased vision, small pupil. Vascular prominence around perimeter of cornea; intraocular tension normal.

Diagnosis: Uveitis, confirmed on slit lamp exam.

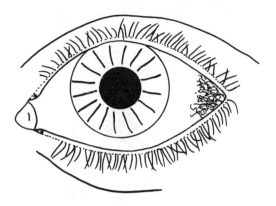

Figure 53. Ocular pain; Blood vessels most prominent temporally.

Diagnosis: Episcleritis. Steroids may be indicated.

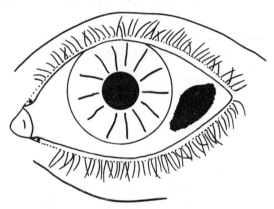

Figure 54. Spontaneously appearing patch of hemorrhage over sclera; painless; vision normal.

Diagnosis: Subconjunctival hemorrhage. No treatment necessary.

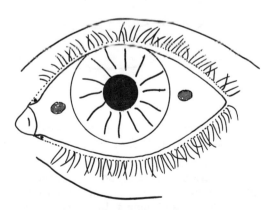

Figure 55. Soft, yellowish patches over sclera at 3 and 9 o'clock positions; patient asymptomatic.

Diagnosis: Pinguecula (a benign condition).

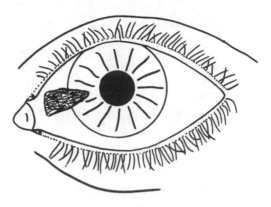

Figure 56. Vascularization extending into the nasal aspect of the cornea; patient asymptomatic.

Diagnosis: Pterygium (a benign condition; may be removed for cosmesis or if it threatens vision by extending too far centrally). The cause is unknown.

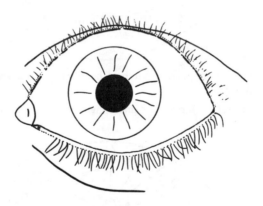

Figure 57. Protruding eye; sclera shows at 12 o'clock position, above the cornea; nervousness; heat intolerance; lid lag on attempted eyelid closure.

Diagnosis: Thyrotoxic exophthalmia. Exophthalmos may also result from a carotid cavernous fistula (abnormal connection between carotid artery and cavernous venous sinus leading to a backup of blood in the orbit), orbital cellulitis, and tumors. In benign hereditary exophthalmos, common in black individuals, the sclera generally does not show at the 12 o'clock position of the cornea.

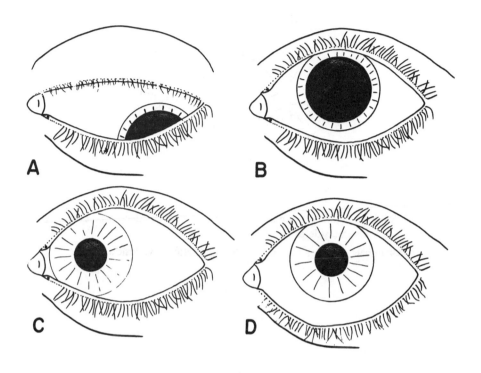

Figure 58. A. Marked ptosis; dilated, fixed pupil; eye turned down and out (left eye).
B. Dilated pupil in one eye, responds slowly to light. No other
abnormality. C. Eye cannot turn outward. Double vision; no other
abnormality. D. Patient cannot close lids; some drooping of lower lid.
Diagnosis: A. Cranial nerve 3 lesion. In CN3 damage secondary to
diabetes, the pupil is commonly spared. B. *Adie's* pupil (tonic pupil), a
benign condition. The pupil in one eye is normally dilated and reacts
slowly to light. There is no ptosis or extraocular muscle weakness. C.
Cranial nerve 6 lesion; no pupillary abnormality. D. Cranial nerve
7 lesion; no pupillary abnormality. Loss of muscle tone causes droopiness
of lower lid.

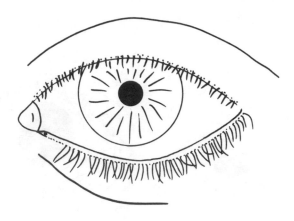

Figure 59. Mild ptosis, miosis (small pupil), and anhydrosis (decreased sweating), all on the same side of the face.

Diagnosis: Horner's syndrome (sympathetic nerve lesion).

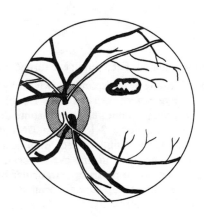

Figure 60. Solitary patch of ragged pigmentation.

Diagnosis: Old inactive chorioretinitis. Cause commonly remains undertermined. Classic causes include toxoplasmosis, syphilis, tuberculosis, sarcoidosis, rubella, histoplasmosis and others. In acute stages the retina and overlying vitreous appear white and hazy.

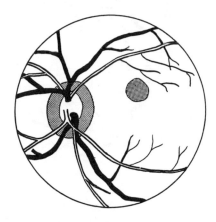

Figure 61. Isolated asymptomatic "freckle", increasing in size over several months.

Diagnosis: Tumor, possible malignant choroidal melanoma. Requires further testing with fluorescein angiography. Malignant melanomas are the most common intraocular malignant tumors, but are particularly rare among black patients. Retinoblastoma is the most common intraocular malignancy in childhood (see p. 37).

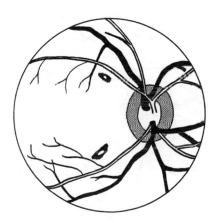

Figure 62. Hemorrhagic areas with whitish centers in a patient with subacute bacterial endocarditis.

Diganosis: Roth spots.

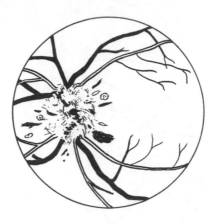

Figure 63. Absent venous pulsations in cup region; blurred disc margins; elevated disc; vessels tourtuous at disc level and difficult to follow completely to the region of the optic cup because of overlying edema; hemorrhages and exudates in the disc region; visual acuity unimpaired.

Diagnosis: Papilledema. If the patient were to have the above, but with marked loss of vision and eye pain, the diagnosis would most likely be papillitis (an inflammation of the disc). If the eye appears normal to viewing and there is marked loss of vision with pain behind the eye, the most likely diagnosis is optic neuritis, in which the inflammation is behind the optic disc, in the optic nerve, and may not be visible.

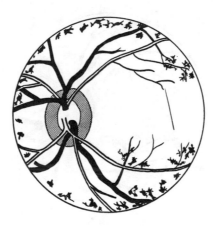

Figure 64. Difficulty seeing at night, "bone-spicule" pigmentary degeneration of the retina in a ring-like distribution.

Diagnosis: Retinitis pigmentosa. Typically, arteriolar narrowing occurs as well (not shown).

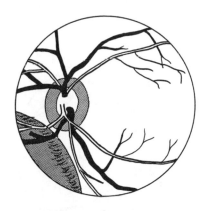

Figure 65. Acute onset of visual loss in the left eye, like "a curtain" drawn partially down over the superotemporal aspect of the visual field.

Diagnosis: Retinal detachment, inferonasal aspect of the left retina.

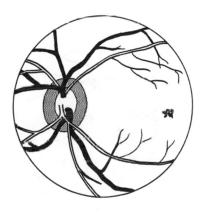

Figure 66. Progressive loss of visual acuity in an elderly patient; lens clear. Pigmentary changes in foveal region.

Diagnosis: Senile macular degeneration.

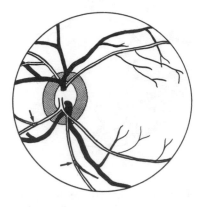

Figure 67. Attacks of *amaurosis fugax* in the right eye and intermittent episodes of weakness on the left side of the body; right carotid bruit; glistening emboli at areas of arteriolar bifurcation (arrows).

Diagnosis: Cholesterol emboli (*Hollenhorst placques)*. Patient is at great risk of developing a stroke.

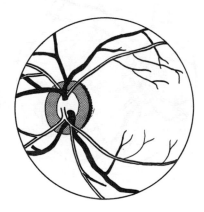

Figure 68. Crescent of pigmentation around the border of the optic disc in a medical student who panicked and thought it reflected a serious condition.

Diagnosis: Benign pigment crescent.

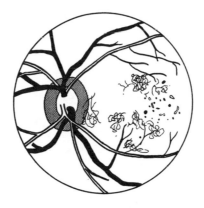

Figure 69. Microaneurysms, "dot" hemorrhages (which may be difficult to distinguish from microaneurysms, that are also present); "blot" hemorrhages, neovascularization, and hard exudates in a diabetic patient.

Diagnosis: Diabetic retinopathy. In hypertensive retinopathy, the hemorrhages tend to be flame-shaped and the exudates soft (cotton wool). See figure 23, 71.

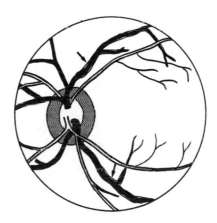

Figure 70. Fuzzy, white discoloration (arrows) surrounding veins.

Diagnosis: Periphlebitis (venous cuffing). This may occur in a variety of inflammations of the retina and choroid. Sometimes the arterioles may be involved (periarteritis). In sarcoid, periphlebitis may have a lardaceous or "candle wax" appearance.

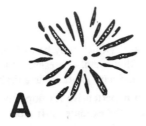 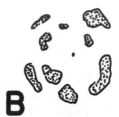

Figure 71. A. Macular star in hypertensive retinopathy. Although exudates in hypertension classically are of the "cotton wool" type, hard exudates may also occur, particularly as seen here, radiating from the fovea.

B. Hard exudates in diabetic retinopathy commonly surround the fovea, as shown here, in "circinate" fashion.

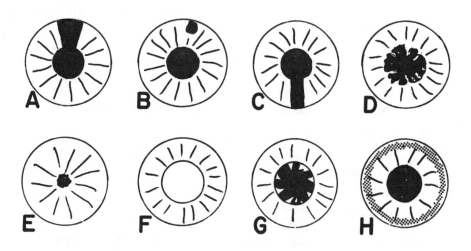

Figure 72. A. "Keyhole pupil" - sector iridectomy, sometimes performed during cataract surgery to insure subsequent adequate drainage of aqueous humor to the anterior chamber (herniating vitreous may otherwise block aqueous flow). It is also performed to allow better post-operative visualization of the retina. B. Peripheral iridectomy. Cosmetically more acceptable than the sector iridectomy; the patient reports less glare. Performed in cataract surgery and also as a primary procedure in angle closure glaucoma, to facilitate aqueous passage to the anterior chamber angle. Sector and peripheral iridectomies are almost always performed in the 12 o'clock position of the iris because the upper lid partially overhangs this region. This allows a better cosmetic result and reduces glare. C. Coloboma of the iris. This embyonic defect occurs in the 6 o'clock position, the site of the embryonic fissure of the eye cup, which does not close properly in colobomas. The retina may be involved with a similar defect. D. Posterior synechiae. The iris sticks to the lens following intraocular inflammation. E. Argyll -Robertson pupil, found in tertiary syphilis. The pupil is characteristically small and irregular and responds to accommodation but not light. F. Dense cataract. This appears white to direct flashlight illumination (but black against a red background, through the ophthalmoscope). G. Peripheral cataract, often associated with good visual acuity. H. Arcus senilis. Grayish, opaque ring close to the periphery of the cornea, associated with aging. In young individuals *(arcus juvenilis)*, it may be associated with hypercholesterolemia.

GLOSSARY

amaurosis fugax - transient loss of vision from retinal ischemia, believed due to vasospasm or obstruction of an arteriole by embolus.

aphakia - absence of lens.

asthenopia - eyestrain (blurred vision, diplopia, headache) from excessive use of the eye.

blepharochalasis - loose overhanging skin fold in upper lid.

Bruch's membrane - the membrane separating the pigment epithelium and choroid.

cataract - lens opacity.

cavernous venous sinus - an important venous drainage area near the brain stem that receives venous outflow from the orbit. The carotid artery and all the nerves entering the orbit run through or near this sinus.

chalazion - inflammation of a meibomian gland.

coloboma - a developmental defect in the closure of the eye cup, leading to a gap in the inferior region of the retina and/or iris.

conjunctiva - the thin transparent vascular membrane overlying the sclera and continuing on the under surface of the lids, in direct apposition to the tear film.

crepitus - crackling sound on palpating skin that contains underlying air.

cycloplegia - paralysis of accommodation.

dermatochalasis - puffiness of skin in the upper lid with aging, commonly due to herniation of orbital fat.

dermatome - the area of skin supplied by one nerve root.

diopter - a unit referring to the converging (plus) or diverging (minus) ability of a lens.

diplopia - double vision.

drusen - small round yellow spots just outside the pigment epithelium, a benign degenerative condition. When in the optic nerve head, drusen appear as bumpy tapioca-like excrescences, which should not be confused with papilledema.

dry-eye syndrome - irritation secondary to decreased tearing, as in Sjogrens syndrome; may be treated with ocular lubricants like methylcellulose (Adsorbotear) and polyvinyl alcohol (Liquifilm tears.) Sometimes, vitamin A ointment may be useful.

episcleritis - inflammation of the connective tissue lying between sclera and conjunctiva.

esotropia - crossed eyes.

exotropia - wall eyes.

fornix - the region where conjunctiva overlying the eye folds back to become the conjunctiva underlying the lid.

fundus - the posterior area of the retina, particularly the area within view of the ophthalmoscope.

Goldmann perimeter - a refined device for plotting visual field defects using lights of varying size and brightness.

hemianopia - loss of vision in half of a visual field.

hemiparesis - weakness of one side of the body.

hypoxia - lack of oxygen.

injection - marked prominence of small vessels.

iridectomy - surgical removal of iris tissue.

keratitis - inflammation of the cornea.

lesion - injury.

limbus - the junction zone between cornea and sclera.

lipemia retinalis - yellow-cream coloring of retinal vessels due to markedly excessive lipids in the blood.

microphthalmia - small eye.

myokymia - twitching of eyelids, a benign transient condition possibly related to fatigue or tension; occurs unilaterally.

neovascularization - formation of new blood vessels.

photophobia - pain on exposure to light.

pinguecula - a benign yellowish, soft, slightly elevated area found nasal or lateral to the cornea, typically nasal.

ptosis - droopy lid.

quadrantopia - loss of vision in one quandrant of a visual field.

sign - what the physician finds, as opposed to a *symptom*.

slit lamp - a specialized microscope for viewing the eye externally and internally; has attachments to alter the size, shape, brightness, and angulation of the light beam, and usually contains a tonometer for measuring intraocular pressure.

stye - an inflamed pimple along the lid margin, representing an infection of a hair follicle or a small local gland.

superior colliculus - the curved roof of the rostral midbrain, associated with various visual reflexes.

symptom - what the patient complains of, as opposed to a *sign*.

synapse - the specialized connection between one nerve cell and another.

synechiae - adhesions secondary to inflammation.

tangent screen - a black screen designed to test for visual field defects by introducing test objects of various sizes in different positions of the visual field.

telangiectasia - an area of excessive numbers of small blood vessels.

trachoma - a chlamydial infection of the eye in which follicles arise in the upper lid conjunctiva, followed by vascular invasion and scarring of the cornea, beginning at its 12 o'clock position.

trichiasis - inward turning of eyelashes against the eye, often causing ocular irritation.

unilateral - present on one side.

vestibular apparatus - the balance-sensing mechanism in the inner ear.

visual field - the extent of what the eye sees when looking forward.

Wilson's disease - a familial disorder of copper metabolism with cirrhosis of the liver and degeneration in the basal ganglia of the brain. Copper deposits in the lens (copper cataracts) and the peripheral cornea, as a greenish-brown ring (Kayser-Fleisher ring).

xerophthalmia - drying and clouding of the cornea with vitamin A deficiency.

INDEX

accommodation, 4, 41
Adie's Pupil, Fig. 58
albinism, 45
alkaptonuria, 45
allergy, 22, 60
amaurosis fugax, 59, glossary, Fig. 67
amblyopia, 16
amyloidosis, 45
anemia, 45
angioid streaks, 46 (see pseudoxanthoma elasticum; sickle cell anemia)
ankylosing spondylitis, 45
anterior chamber, 2, 54
aqueous humor, 2
arcus juvenilis, Fig. 72
Argyll-Robertson pupil, 41, Fig. 72
arteriovenous nicking, 34
artery
    central retinal, 6, 59
    ophthalmic, 8
asthenopia, 60
astigmatism, 14
atopic dermatitis, 45
band keratopathy, 45, 46
Behcet's syndrome, 45
Bell's palsy, 42, Fig. 58
blepharitis, 22, Fig. 49
belpharochalasis, glossary
Bowman's membrane, 3
carcinoma, basal cell, 22, Fig. 40
cataract, 5, 21, 37, 57, Fig. 72
cavernous venous sinus, 22
cellulitis, 22
chalazion, 9, 22, Fig. 39
chemical burns, 31
chorioretinitis, 6, Fig. 60
choroid, 5
ciliary body, 2
cluster headache, 44
coloboma, Fig. 72
color vision, 19
conjunctiva, 8
conjunctivitis, 23, 60, Fig. 50
    gonococcal, 23
    inclusion, 24
    silver nitrate induced, 24
contact lenses, 2, 20

contact lens syndrome, 24
copper wiring, 33
cornea, 2, 24
corneal transplantation, 31
cystic fibrosis, 45
cystinosis, 45
cytomegalic inclusion disease, 45
dacryoadenitis, 23, Fig. 44
dacryocystitis, 23, Fig. 45
dermatochalasis, glossary
dermatomyositis, 45
Descemet's membrane, 3
diabetes, 27, 34, 45
Diamox (acetazolamide), 28
Down's syndrome, 45
drusen, glossary
dry eye syndrome, glossary
ectropion, Fig. 42
Ehlers-Danlos syndrome, 45
entropion, Fig. 43
epicanthal folds, 19
epinephrine, in glaucoma, 28
episcleritis, 24, 60, Fig. 53
floaters, 59
fluorescein angiography, 36, 37
foreign body, removal, 55
fornix, 8
fovea, 36, 39
Freidrich's ataxia, 45
galactosemia, 45
gland
    lacrimal, 9
    meibomian, 2
glaucoma, 4, 25, 31, 38, 39
    narrow angle, 25, Fig. 51
    open angle, 26, 35
glomerulonephritis, 45
Goldmann perimeter, 27
goniolens, 55
gout, 45
hemorrhage, arterial, 33, 59
hemorrhage subconjunctival, 23, Fig. 54
hemorrhage, venous, 34, 59
hereditary hemorrhagic telangiectasia, 45
herpes simplex, 24, Fig. 47

herpes zoster, 45
histoplasmosis, 45
Hollenhorst plaques, Fig. 67
homocystinuria, 45
Horner's syndrome, Fig. 59
hyperlipidemia, 45
hyperopia, 10
hyperparathyroidism, 45
hypertensive retinopathy, 33
hyperthyroidism, 45, Fig. 57
hyphema, 30, Fig. 48
hypoparathyroidism, 45
hypopyon, 30
hypothyroidism, 46
internuclear ophthalmoplegia, 42
iridectomy, Fig. 72
iris, 2
keratitis, 46
keratoconus, 20
kernicterus, 46
lacrimal puncta, 9
lacrimal sac, 9
laser photocoagulation
    in diabetes, 34
    in glaucoma, 28
lead poisoning, 46
lens, 2
lens implant, 21
lipemia retinalis, in hyperlipidemia, 45
lupus erythematosis, 46
macroglobulinemia, 46
macular degeneration, 36, Fig. 66
macular star, Fig. 71
Marchesani syndrome, 46
Marfan's syndrome, 46
marijuana, in glaucoma therapy, 28
medial longitudinal fasciculus, 41
melanoma, 36, Fig. 61
microaneurysms, 34, Fig. 69
migraine, 43, 46, 59
mucopolysaccharidoses, 46
multiple sclerosis, 38, 46
muscles, extraocular, 6, 7
    inferior oblique, 7
    lateral rectus, 7
    levator palpebrae superioris, 7, 9

medial rectus, 7
Muller's, 7
orbicularis, 7, 9
superior oblique, 7
superior rectus, 7
muscles, intraocular,
of ciliary body, 3
of iris, 4
myasthenia gravis, 46
myokymia, glossary
myopia, 10
myotonia, 46
neovascularization, of retina,
    34, Fig. 69
nerve
        abducens (CN6), 8
        facial (CN7), 42
        infraorbital, 30
        oculomotor (CN3), 8
        optic (CN2), 8
        sympathetics, 8
        trigeminal (CN5), 43
        trochlear (CN4), 8
neurofibromatosis, 46
nystagmus, 42
ophthalmoscope
    direct, 49
    indirect, 52
optic disc, 26
osteogenesis imperfecta, 46
papilledema, 35, 36, Fig. 63
papillitis, 35, 36
Parinaud's syndrome, 42
periphlebitis, Fig. 70
phospholine iodide, 16, 28
photophobia, 60
photoreceptors, 5
pigment epithelium, 5
pilocarpine, 26, 28
pinguecula, Fig. 55
pinhole effect, 10
polyarteritis nodosa, 46
polycythemia, 46
posterior chamber, 2
presbyopia, 12
pseudostrabismus, 18

pseudoxanthoma elasticum, 46
pterygium, Fig. 56
ptosis, Figs. 58, 59
pupil, 2
pupillary reflex, 40
radial keratotomy, 21
radiation exposure, 46
refraction, 2, 10
Reiter's syndrome, 46
retina, 5
    detachment, 6, 36, 59, Fig. 65
    hemorrhage, 31
retinitis pigmentosa, 37, 60, Fig. 64
retinoblastoma, 37
retrolental fibroplasia, 37
rheumatoid arthritis, 46
Riley-Day syndrome, 46
rosacea, 46
Rosenbaum card, 11
Roth spots, Fig. 62
rubella, 46
sarcoid, 46
Schlemm's canal, 2, 25
sclera, 5
scleritis, 24, 60
sickle cell anemia, 46
silver wiring, 33
Sjogren's syndrome, 47
slit lamp, 57
Snellen chart, 10
stereoscopic vision, 19
Stevens-Johnson syndrome, 47
strabismus, 16

Sturge-Weber disease, 47
stye, 9, 22, Fig. 38
subacute bacterial endocarditis, 47
sympathetic ophthalmia, 31
syphilis, 47
tangent screen, glossary
tarsal plate, 9
Tay-Sachs disease, 47
tear film, 9
temporal arteritis, 44, 47
tonometry, 25, 53
toxemia, 47
toxoplasmosis, 47
trachoma, 24, 35
transient ischemic
    attack, 59
trichinosis, 47
tuberculosis, 47
tuberous sclerosis, 47
ulcerative colitis, 47
uvea, 6
uveitis, 6, 29, Fig. 52
vein, hemorrhage, 34, 59
vein, ophthalmic, 8
vitamin deficiency, 47
vitreous chamber, 2
Von-Hippel Lindau disease, 47
Wilm's tumor, 47
Wilson's disease, 4, 47
xanthelasma, 22, Fig. 41
xerophthalmia, 47
zonules, 4

NOTES

NOTES

NOTES

NOTES

NOTES

NOTES

NOTES